The Neural Foundation of Experience

The Role of Vibrating Neurons

by

David LaBerge, University of California, Irvine

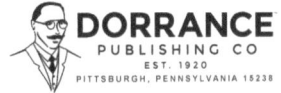

DORRANCE
PUBLISHING CO
EST. 1920
PITTSBURGH, PENNSYLVANIA 15238

Dorrance Publishing Co
585 Alpha Drive
Pittsburgh, PA 15238
Visit our website at *www.dorrancebookstore.com*

ISBN: 978-1-6470-2559-5
eISBN: 978-1-6470-2669-1

This book is dedicated to
the students and faculty of Bard College at Simon's Rock.

ALSO BY DAVID LABERGE

Attentional Processing: The Brain's Art of Mindfulness
Harvard University Press

Acknowledgments

After I retired from the University of California, Irvine in 1997, I moved to Great Barrington, Massachusetts to teach cognitive neuroscience at Simon's Rock College (now named Bard College at Simon's Rock), where my wife, Jan Lawry, was Associate Dean. Simon's Rock is an early college that enrolls gifted students after their second year of high school. In classes of about 15, these very bright young students reacted in fresh and challenging ways to new ideas about the workings of the brain that I was developing at the time. I am very grateful for the informative and lively ways that they bounced ideas to each other and back to me, and I believe that the eventual shape of many concepts in this book came from those classes.

During my years at Simon's Rock I audited several courses taught by the faculty, and the courses in electronics and poetry provided fertile backgrounds for material in several chapters of this book. About halfway through my decade at Simon's Rock, I met a physicist who lived near the college, and he began to audit my courses. A year later Ray Kasevich and I began having weekly meetings at his office to discuss the electrical aspects of neurons. Those discussions eventually led to four co-authored publications on the topic of the apical dendrites of neurons. This book owes much to him for his sharing with me his expertise in electrical physics.

I am also indebted to Anne O'Dwyer, Professor of Psychology Simon's Rock College, for using an early draft of this book as the text in a tutorial class in neuroscience. When I periodically asked about the reactions of the students to the book, the answer was always the same: "The students love this book."

I thank Ray Kasevich, Anne LaBerge , Edward Lawry, and Sandra Wu for reading an early draft of this book and offering helpful comments. I thank Anne LaBerge for her ideas about the resonant dendrite in music and for her demonstrations with the flute how this vibrating part of a neuron works. To Anne O'Dwyer and Sandra Wu go my special thanks for their many improvements in the presentation of the ideas in the text. Any errors in the ideas or the writing are my own. Also I thank Sandra Kruse of Dorrance Publishing for guiding me smoothly through the preparation of the manuscript for publication.

To my wife, Jan Lawry, goes very special thanks, not only for her contribution to the organizing of several early drafts of the manuscript and to the choosing of the book's title, but also for two years of putting up with someone whose mind was often somewhere else, chasing the apical dendrite.

Introduction

I bring to the writing of this book over 40 years of research and teaching in major universities, the most recent being the University of California, Irvine. The last 8 of my 75 publications are about the workings of a neural fiber called the apical dendrite — the central idea of this book and the hero of this story about the brain.

This book is about neurons in the brain, and how some neurons make it possible for us to *think* about eating an apple, and other neurons enable us to *enjoy* eating an apple.

Most of us are familiar with the "thinking" neurons because they are like the "information-in and information-out" devices of a computer. But, unlike the computer, our brains also contain many neurons which enable us to enjoy colorful sunsets, the sounds of music, and the presence of friends and family.

The neurons that enable us to enjoy and savor the world vibrate electrically instead of processing information. The part of the neuron that produces vibrations is called the *apical dendrite*, which is a very long fiber that extends upward from the center of the neuron. It is the place in the brain where psychology, biology, and physics meet.

Neurons that vibrate provide our minds with more than subjective experiences of sensations and feelings. They decide which neurons can communicate with each other, and they provide an internal "clock" that determines exactly when each neuron will send its output to another neuron. Both of these features are necessary for processing information. In addition, the ability of vibrating neurons to control the intensity and duration of a mental state provides a basis for attention, and potentially a basis for consciousness.

In the writing of this book I have tried to avoid technical language wherever possible and I use many illustrations so that readers can easily understand the new ideas whether or not they have a background in biology, psychology, or neuroscience. The inclusion of many illustrations is intended to gradually develop the more challenging concepts so readers can "see" how neurons work together in circuits. It is my hope that the ideas presented here will encourage a greater curiosity and appreciation for our brains and all that they make possible for us.

Contents

Chapter 1. Is Your Brain a Computer? 1

Chapter 2. When Does the Brain Act Like a Computer? 3

Chapter 3. Is Mental Life More Than Processing Information? 11

Chapter 4. How the Vibrating Apical Dendrite Works 27

Chapter 5. The Two Neural Systems of Mental Life: A Brief Summary . .37

Chapter 6. The Role of the Apical Dendrite in Attention 47

Chapter 7. The Learning of Familiarity and Skills 69

Chapter 8. How Does the Brain Produce an Intense Experience? 91

Chapter 9. The Role of the Insula in the Experiencing of Feelings 105

Chapter 10. Being on the Same Wavelength 119

Chapter 11. Consciousness. 147

Chapter 12. Conclusions and Summary 155

Chapter 1

Is Your Brain a Computer?

Computers are amazing. They can do much of our thinking for us. They correct our spelling errors and show us where our sentences have lumpy grammar. They can solve complex mathematics problems in less than a second. As they got smaller in size over the past decade, they got smarter and faster. As I write this book, there are computers that can sift through in seconds the amount of data it would take months or even years for a human to sift through. While we are driving our car, a computer can instantly pinpoint our location on the dashboard display. They alert us to upcoming traffic conditions and can answer our routine questions for information. They give their answers promptly and later if we ask the same question again, the voice does not begin with "As I told you before," but cheerfully repeats the answer, all in a friendly voice that sometimes annoys our spouses. A computer can even drive our car for us while we take a cat nap.

Larger computers design clothing and even design new computers. Our grocery store can track our buying habits and mail us coupons that discount our favorite purchases. For the student who wants to write a paper about the effect of exercise on mental concentration the computer can help out by doing a quick search of what is currently known about the topic. The computers can get information from a giant computer "library in the cloud" faster than we can say "library in the cloud." Always obedient, our computers open a world of information for us, right at our fingertips.

Because computers do so many things that our brains do, we cannot help wondering if someday they can take the next big step toward what it means to be human—what we humans all do every day with the help of our human brains: Could computers eventually experience sensations of color, musical tunes, and feelings of fear and joy?

This book tries to answer this question by looking inside the computer and inside the brain and then comparing the ways that each one works. Doing this may seem like a huge undertaking, fraught with technical details understood only by experts. But it turns out that recent discoveries in neuroscience now make it possible not only to see how computers and brains are alike, but also, and perhaps more importantly, easily understand things the brain can do that computers cannot do. Rather than relying on technical explanations used in textbooks and research articles, this book relies on simple drawings and familiar metaphors to ease the reader's journey to understanding a new view of the workings of the brain.

Chapter 2

When Does the Brain Act Like a Computer

The picture shown in Figure 2.1 shows a person gazing at a mountain[1]. What do you think is happening in his brain while he looks at that mountain? You might answer that his brain is processing something that the eyes are sending to it. When asked what this "something" is, you might reply that it is like what happens when a digital camera sends a message from the camera screen to a storage chip in the camera. So far, so good. But what is that message made of?

The message that the screen of a camera sends to its storage chip is a string of electric pulses and spaces. Pulses and spaces move along a wire with an even rhythm, like marching to a drum-beat. We can write a string of pulses as 1's and 0's, in which 1's are pulses and 0's are spaces or pauses, for example, 11010001101. Each 1 is an electric pulse, and each 0 is a space (or no-pulse). Each 1 or 0 counts as one bit of information.

It will help to go over these basic ideas again in preparation for comparing the brain with a computer. This chapter aims to make clear how the computer and the brain are similar and how they are different. If the brain were wired like a computer it might be drawn something like the diagram in Figure 2.2. This picture is a simplified drawing of a computer circuit board, showing the wires that connect small pads. The

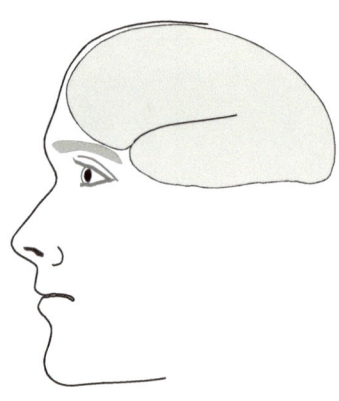

Figure 2.1

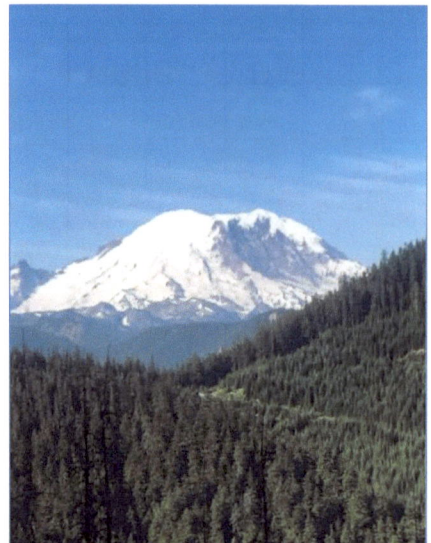

Figure 2.1

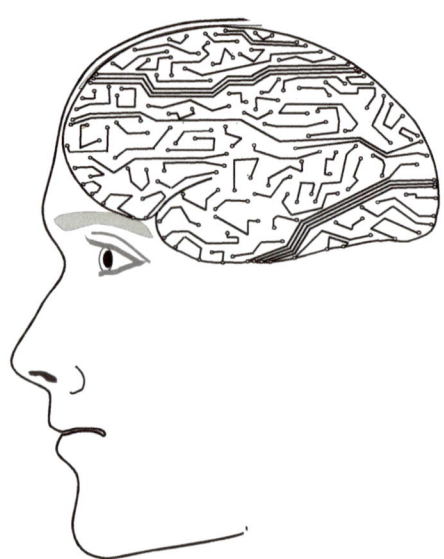

Figure 2.2

Figure 2.2

pads, shown here as small circles, are points where tiny electronic de-vices are attached, and sometimes a pad connects a device to a circuit on the opposite side of the thin circuit board. A larger picture of both the lines and the electronic devices would look like a small city with many streets with a building sitting in the intersection of each street, instead of on one of the street corners.

The feature of the circuit board that is most helpful in comparing the computer to the brain is the grid-like map of connections between pads. The grid resembles a large wire mesh, which is a material widely used for fencing and cages. Figure 2.3 shows the grid of the circuit board of a laptop computer. The circuit board of a computer is designed by placing an electronic device at some of the intersections of grid lines and then connecting the devices to each other with tiny wires mapped on the grid. The result is a map showing the routes that electric pulses can take during the processing of bits of information. This routing map makes it clear that computation, the basic activity of a computer, con-sists of moving bits of information from one place to another. Since all circuit boards are constructed upon the grid, the simple diagram of a bare grid can serve as the symbol of a circuit board, as shown in Figure 2.3 (bottom right).

The diagram in Figure 2.4 shows that connections of neurons in the brain can also be viewed as having a grid-like structure. This picture shows a thin grid that is spread out beneath the surface of the brain. Each point where one line crosses another line represents the place where a neuron could be located, and each neuron resembles a pad on a circuit board where a processing device could be attached. Therefore, the outer covering of the brain is the place to look for the neural activ-ities that most resemble the activities of a computer.

Building on this foundation, the left side of Figure 2.5 shows the layout of neurons in a micro-photograph of some of the neurons lo-cated in a layer near the surface of the brain. The right side of Figure 2.5 identifies the main parts of a neuron. A neuron can have hundreds

Network Grid Inside a Laptop Computer

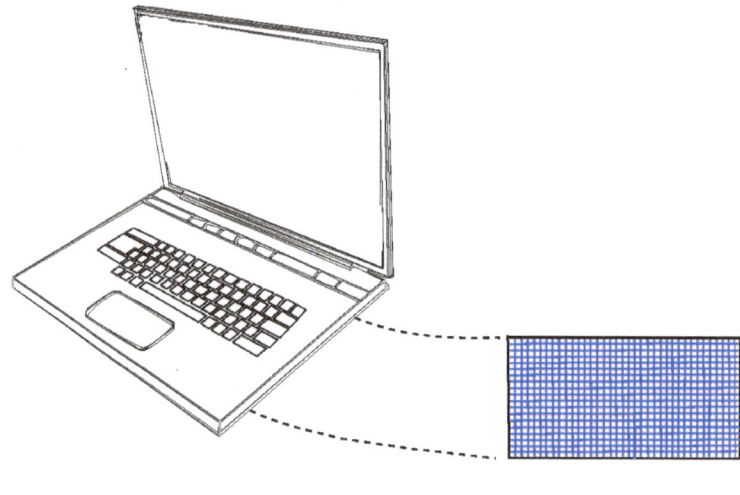

Figure 2.3

Figure 2.4

The Thin Network Grid Located
Near the Surface of the Brain

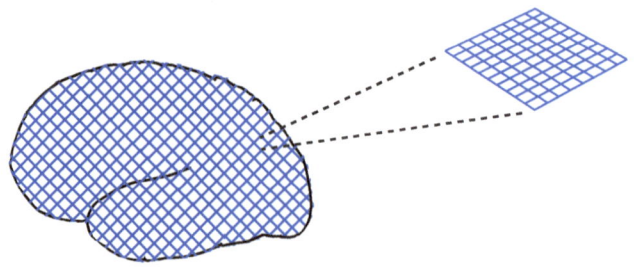

Figure 2.4

of inputs that contact the surfaces of its dendrites, but there is one out-put fiber, the axon, and this fiber is very thin and often very long.

The neuron's electric pulse signal is a very brief spike of voltage that peaks at the same level of intensity, or else there is no spike at all. This "all-or-nothing" feature of the computer signal is like the "on-or-off" feature of the basic computer signal which, as shown earlier, can be coded as a 1 or a 0. The neuron receives electric pulses from other neurons and processes these inputs into a single train of pulses in the axon. The axon often branches out and sends duplicate signals to many other neurons. Sometimes the axon is very long, extending from the brain to a point in the spinal cord, or extending from the spinal cord to the tip of a toe or to the end of a fin. As you might imagine, giraffes and whales have the longest axon fibers in mammals.

Figure 2.6 illustrates electric spikes on a neural axon and electric pulses on a computer wire and on a telegraph wire. This figure shows that the electric activity of all three transmission systems use an on-or-off type of signal to transmit information from one place to another place within their systems.

The electric signal that is sent along an axon fiber typicallly con-tains less energy than the electric signal that is sent along computer wire. The voltage intensity of the square pulse in a typical computer is about five volts above a baseline of zero volts, and the voltage of a spike of a typical neuron is usually about 100 millivolts (100 x 1/1000 of a volt) between its baseline and its peak. So the voltage intensity of a typi-cal neural pulse is about 1/50 the voltage of a typical computer pulse. Apparently the electric pulses sent by neurons contain much lower en-ergy than the electric pulses sent along wires of computers.

Returning to the example of light from a mountain scene striking the eye, the eye converts the light to electric spike pulses and sends those spikes to the brain, where they enter a network of neurons that both receive the spike information and process it into its own series of spikes. This event is illustrated in Figure 2.7 where spike pulses enter

A Network of Neurons

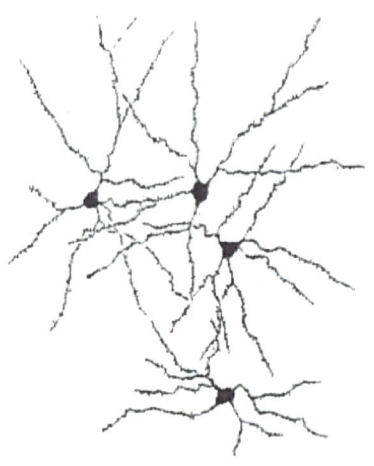

The Neuron and Its Parts

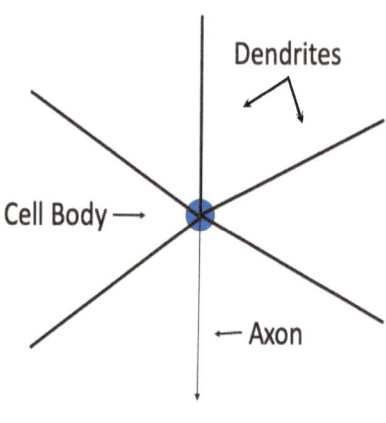

Dendrites

Cell Body ⟶

⟵ Axon

Figure 2.5

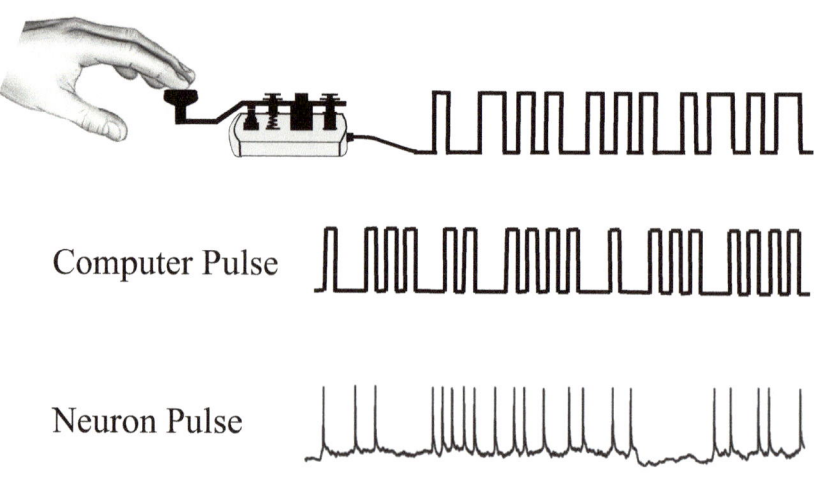

Computer Pulse

Neuron Pulse

Figure 2.6

part of a network grid in the brain. The processing route taken by a series of pulses in a computer is given by the instructions of the computer program, but the specific route taken by a train of spikes in the brain is determined by genetics and what was learned from past experiences of seeing an object. Each neuron acts like a switch that guides a train of spikes into the pathway or pathways the spike information will take when it leaves the neuron.

Is moving spikes from place to place all that the neurons do in the brain? Could there be "something else" that neurons also do to produce our mental life? This is a shocking thought for many people who have learned about the workings of the brain in the context of the computer model. If there really is something going on in the brain besides processing information, what is it? This is the central question of this book that we will be exploring over the remaining chapters.

Network Circuit

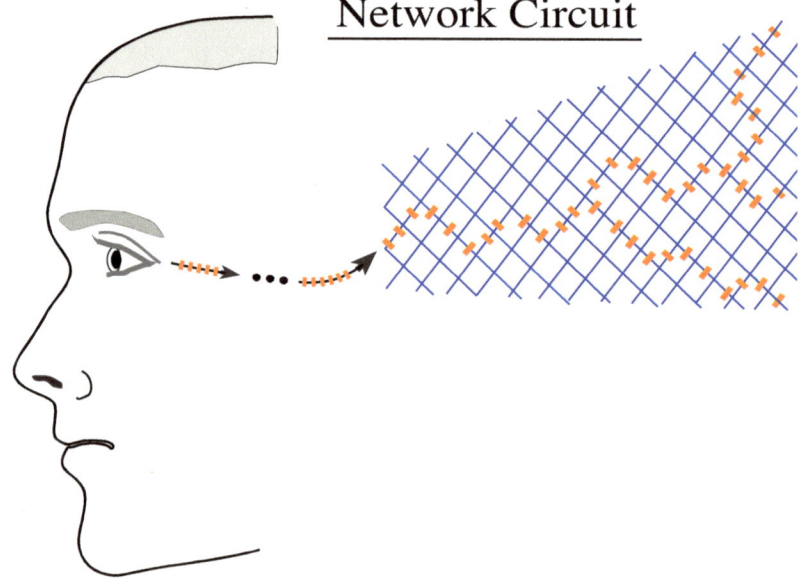

Figure 2.7

Chapter 3

Is Mental LIfe More
Than Processing Information?

Many people, including many scientists, believe that someday networks of computers will be able to produce the sensations of the color and taste of an apple, the sound of a bell, and the feelings of joy and fear. With the right hardware and software, they say, future computers will be able to add *sentience*, the sensations and feelings of our mental life, to the thinking, speaking, and moving of limbs that computer robots already can do.

Instead of looking for ways that a human brain could use computer-like networks of connected neurons to produce feelings and sensations, this book examines a neural fiber that acts differently than the wires that make up a computer network grid. Recalling the descriptions of neural fibers in Chapter 2, dendrite fibers receive electric spikes sent from other neurons, while axon fibers send electric spikes to other neurons. Figure 2.5 (right side) illustrates these two major types of fibers within a neuron that resembles the drawing typically found in text-books. As the story of the third kind of fiber unfolds, it will be revealed that this fiber provides our mental life with more things than sensations and feelings, things that were not anticipated when I began to investigate this fiber 20 years ago.

This special neural fiber is called the apical dendrite, and it is shown in Figure 3.1, where it forms the top part (apex) of the larger neuron shown on the right side of this figure. The drawings of the two neurons in Figure 3.1 were made by a neuroscientist[1] while looking through a high-powered microscope.

The apical dendrite is not "just another dendrite" that receives input pulses from other neurons, like the dendrites of the neuron shown on the left side of Figure 3.1 and the neurons in Figure 2.5. The unusual length of the apical dendrite shown on the right side of Figure 3.1 sets this neuron apart from all other kinds of neurons in the brain. The name of the neuron that contains an apical dendrite that is longer than its other dendrites is called a *pyramidal neuron* because of the pyramid-like shape of its cell body (to see how this neuron is usually drawn look ahead to Figure 3.3). The typical shape of other kinds of neurons is shown in Figure 2.5 and on the left side of Figure 3.1. When the top dendrite is the same size as the other dendrites, the neuron is called a stellate (star-like) neuron, and when the top dendrite is longer than the other dendrites the neuron is called a pyramidal neuron. The star-like appearance of the stellate neuron closely resembles the shape of the most common neurons in the spinal cord of mammals. It is the shape of the model neuron found in most of the introductory textbooks of biology and psychology, where it is used to describe the basic structure and function of a neuron. A closer examination of Figure 3.1 reveals that there is more than the shape of the pyramidal neuron's cell body that gives it a different appearance than the stellate neuron. The two neurons also differ in the thickness of the shaft of the top dendrite and in the size of the cell body.

Looking at the two neurons shown in Figure 3.1, one could imagine that the pyramidal neuron could easily be made from the stellate neuron by grabbing the dendrite at the top of the cell body and pulling on

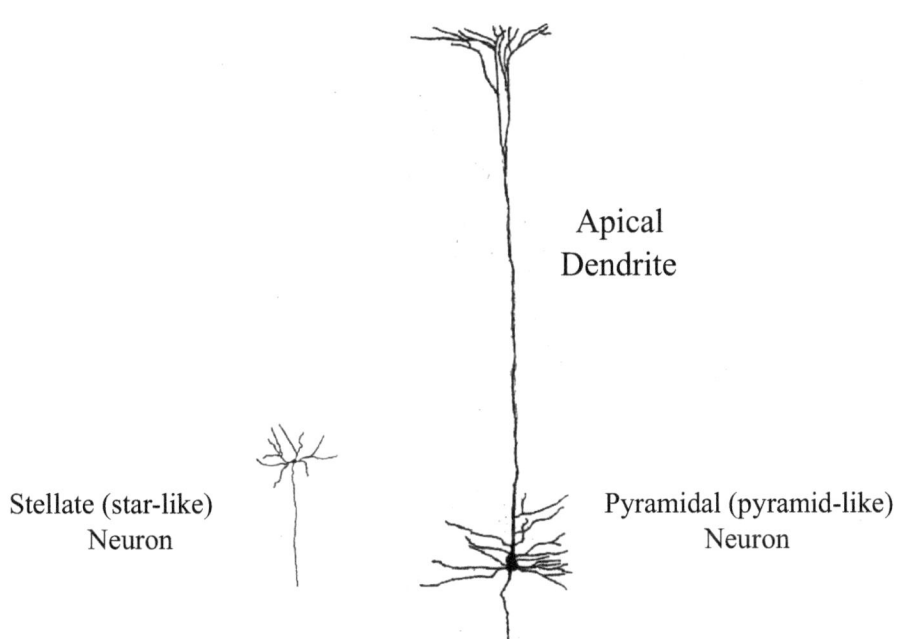

Stellate (star-like)
Neuron

Apical
Dendrite

Pyramidal (pyramid-like)
Neuron

Figure 3.1

it to make it longer. The large difference between the top dendrite of the stellate neuron and the pyramidal neuron suggests that the increase in length of the apical dendrite must have gone through stages in genetic history when the apical dendrite may have had shorter lengths.

It appears that the evolutionary appearance of this single long dendrite at the top of many cortical neurons marks the transition from a species whose brain activity is dominated by simple spinal cord neurons to a new kind of species, a species whose brain activity would eventually be dominated by this neuron with its long apical dendrite.

The genetic history of the length of the apical dendrites of mammals is shown in Figure 3.2. This figure shows the typical length of the apical dendrite for five species of mammals[2].

Apical dendrites are usually either long or short. The short apical dendrite has an important role in mental life, which will be examined later in a Chapter 10. For now, the important observation of Figure 3.2 is the steady increase in the length of the long apical dendrite as the mammal advances from mouse to human. Could these remarkable differences in the length of the apical dendrite suggest what it would be like to be a mouse or a cat?

Now that we know that pyramidal neurons, with their long apical dendrites, are a dominant characteristic of monkeys and humans, one might ask another question: "Are there enough pyramidal neurons in the brain to enable their apical dendrites to influence the ways we see, hear, and feel in a typical day of our life?" The simple image of a dime can help to visualize the number of pyramidal neurons packed into the brain.

When a thin slice of the brain is examined under a high-powered microscope the pyramidal neuron stands out because its cell body is larger and its apical dendrite is thicker and longer than the dendrites of most other neurons. These features of the pyramidal neuron make them relatively easy to count when looking through the microscope.

What researchers have found[3] can be summarized in this easy way. If a dime is placed anywhere on the head over the brain the number of

Long and Short Apical Dendrites
In Five Species of Mammals

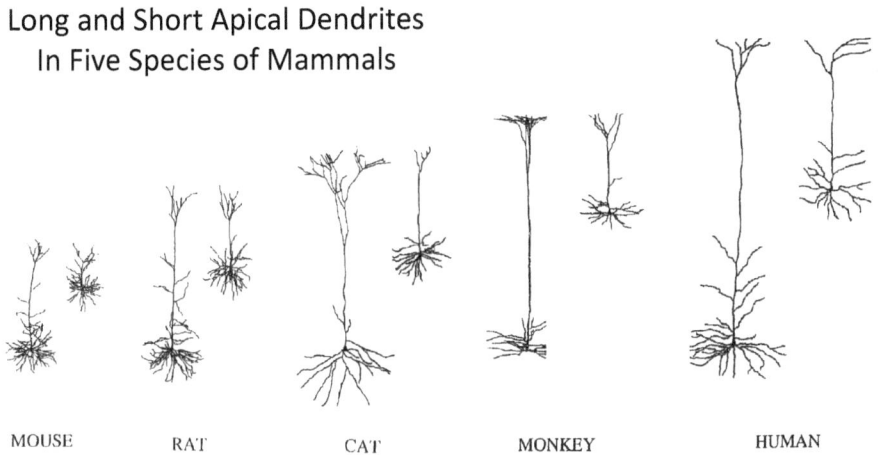

MOUSE   RAT   CAT   MONKEY   HUMAN

Figure 3.2

neurons of all kinds that lie in the cortex (the outer layer of the brain) directly underneath the dime is about 30,000,000 neurons (in the primary visual area at the back of the brain the estimated number of neurons under a dime is up to 2.5 times greater than that of other areas of the cortex). Of the 30,000,000 neurons about 20,000,000 are pyramidal neurons, each with its one apical dendrite. About 5,000,000 of these pyramidal neurons have a long apical dendrite and about 15,000,000 have a short apical dendrite (see Figure 3.2). When you imagine so many neurons under the area of a dime, you can begin to imagine the incredibly small size of a pyramidal neuron. The sizes of almost all other types of neurons are even smaller.

Therefore, the most common neuron in the brain's cortex, where mental activity takes place, is the pyramidal neuron. So, it would seem that the model neuron for the brain's mental or cognitive activity should be the pyramidal neuron, not the stellate neuron. Figure 3.3 shows a diagram of the pyramidal neuron identifying its important parts. Comparing the neuron in Figure 3.3 with the standard neuron in Figure 2.5 reveals that they are very similar in structure, especially in animals toward the bottom of the mammalian scale. Stellate neurons make up about 5% of the neurons in the cortex (the outer layer of the brain), while pyramidal neurons make up about 80% of the cortical neurons.

The two kinds of neurons show their different ways of doing their electric work in Figure 3.4. The stellate neuron, whose dendrites are of similar lengths is part of a network circuit, and the long pyramidal neuron, whose top dendrite is much longer than the other dendrites, is part of a loop circuit. The short pyramidal neuron and its circuitry will be described in detail later in Chapter 10.

Figure 3.4 shows that the thalamus is the first location in the brain where a chain of pulses from the eye diverge and enter the network and loop circuits. In a network, pulses move from one place to another place, but in a loop, pulses stay in the loop and keep moving around it. The diagram in Fibure 3.4 showing the separation of pulse movements

Parts of a Neuron

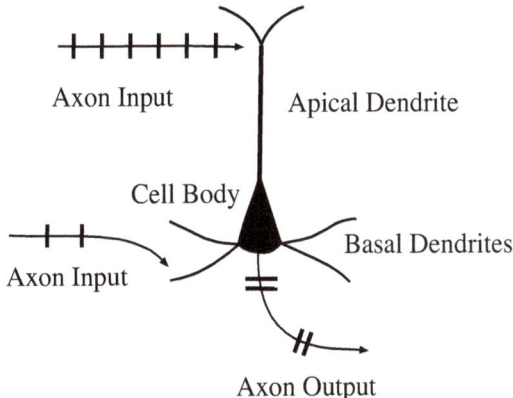

Axon Input

Apical Dendrite

Cell Body

Axon Input

Basal Dendrites

Axon Output

| Electric Pulse

Figure 3.3

Network and Loop Circuits

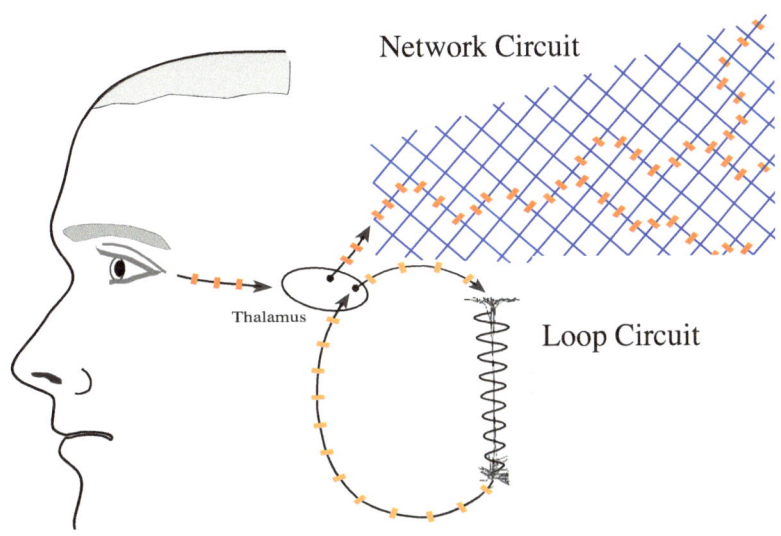

Network Circuit

Thalamus

Loop Circuit

Figure 3.4

into network and loop circuits is presumed to be the same for hearing, touch, smell, and taste.

It is important to point out that the circuit in Figure 3.4 that contains the apical dendrite also contains the thalamus. The thalamus is about the size of a robin's egg and is located near the center of the brain (see Figure 3.5), which is emblematic of its importance in mental activity. The word *thalamus* (a Latin word meaning inner chamber or bridal chamber) is one of the few anatomical structures introduced in this book, but it will have a central role in much of our later descriptions of brain activities.

Students of biology or psychology courses may remember that the thalamus serves as a relay station between the senses and the brain's cortex (the cerebral cortex is the outer layer of the brain where most of mental processing takes place). For example, we already know that neural pulses from the eyes contact the thalamus on their way to the visual area of the cortex, and pulses from the ears and skin surfaces do the same. The word "relay" means to receive and pass on something. But as research revealed more about the workings of the thalamus, neuroscientists began to suspect that the thalamus does more than simply pass on information like a relay runner passes on the baton to the next runner in a race. Some early researchers of the thalamus were reminded that the French word "relais" has the same pronunciation as the word "relay," but relais means an inn or a resort where a traveler remains for a time and does things other than taking a short break before getting back on the road, such as spending the night in the (probably not very restful) thalamic bed.

The new question is: What else is the thalamus doing in addition to passing along information from the senses to the cortex? For one thing, when the thalamus relays signals to the cortex of the brain, it receives messages by a returning fiber from the same cortical neuron that the thalamic fiber had initially targeted. In other words, the thalamus is connected to the cortex by many loop circuits. Furthermore, studies

The Thalamus in the Brain

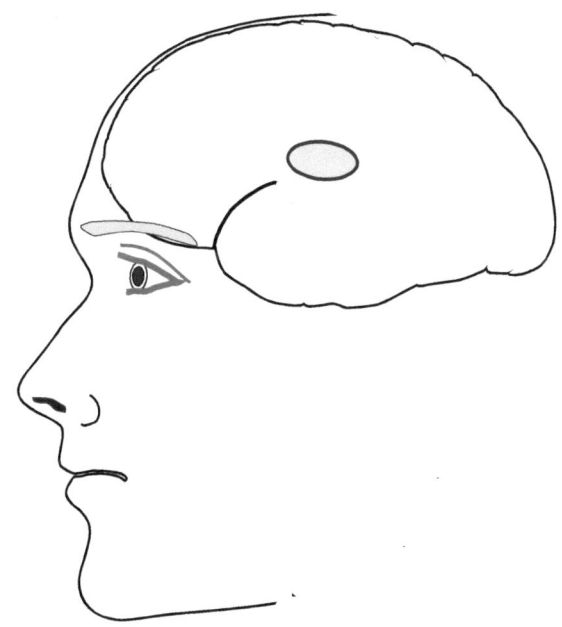

Figure 3.5

of neural connections between the thalamus and cortex have found that for every fiber sent to the cortex the thalamus receives about 10 axon fibers from the cortex. This anatomical observation at first seemed very puzzling in view of the common belief that the role of the thalamus is to move information from the senses to the cortex. Why are so many fibers returning information from the cortex to the thalamus? It seems that many thalamus-to-cortex fibers branch out and connect with several pyramidal neurons, and each of these neurons returns an axon fiber to the thalamus.

Bearing in mind that a major role of the thalamus is to send neural fibers to the cortex, it will be easier to understand how the pyramidal neuron and its apical dendrite operate from the larger context of the whole brain. Figure 3.6 shows a cutaway view of the brain that reveals the interior of the brain and its outside layer. As mentioned before, the outside layer is called the cortex and it is sometimes called "grey matter" because the cell bodies and dendrites inside it have no insulating covering, so their color is grey. The white region is called "white matter" because it contains the long axons that are covered by white myelin insulation.

The drawings in Figure 3.7 show what happens inside the apical dendrite when it is active. When it receives pulses from the thalamus (see the upper part of the loop at Figure 3.7A), the dendrite becomes electrically active. This electric activity consists of surges of current (see Figure 3.7B), but the surges are not strong enough to produce electric spikes. This low-voltage feature of the apical dendrite clearly sets it apart from axon fibers in the neural network, which carry spikes of high voltage that penetrate the membrane and spread to the outside of the axon fiber.

The surge of current is a bunching up of positive electric charges, somewhat like runners in a race that sometimes run in groups that are separated by a short distance. The third drawing of the pyramidal neuron (see Figure 3.7C) shows the electric result of a series of surges moving down the apical dendrite. Each surge of current shifts the charge

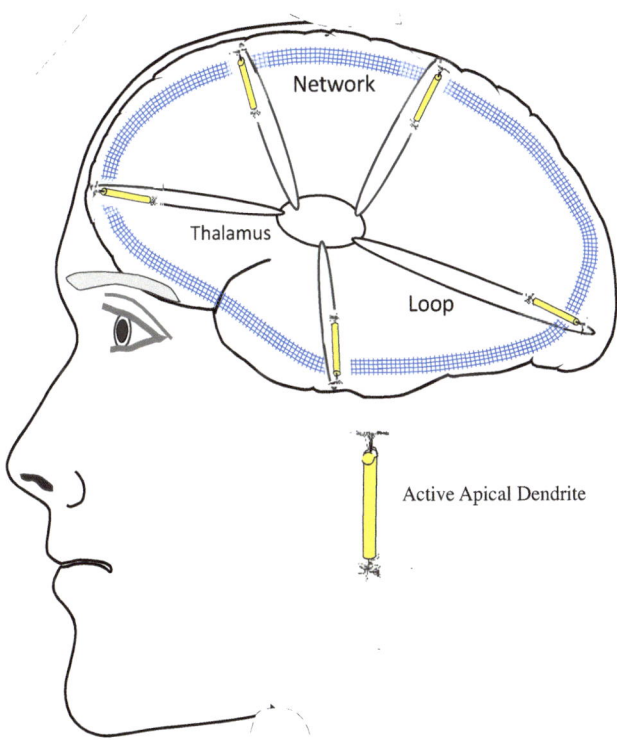

Network

Thalamus

Loop

Active Apical Dendrite

Figure 3.6

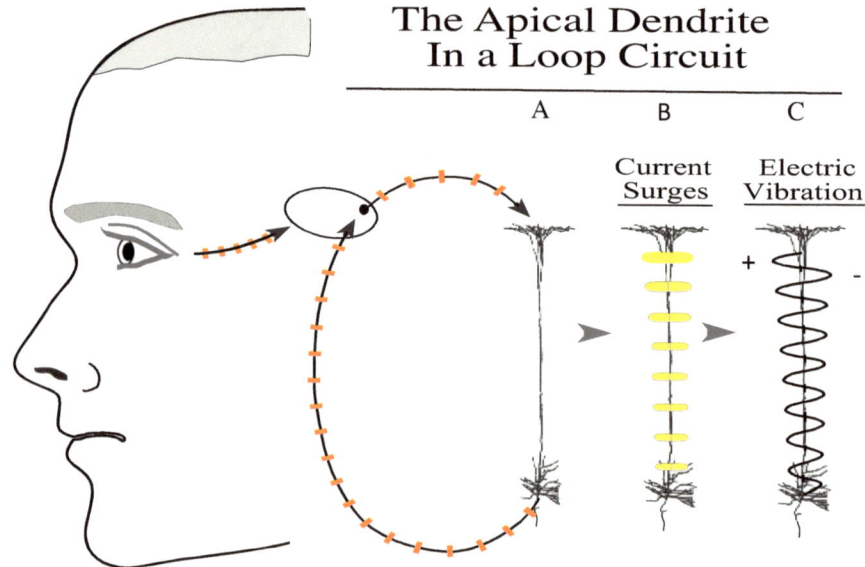

Figure 3.7

of the electric field that surrounds a surge to positive and the charge of the field surrounding a gap between surges to negative, which is represented by the plus-to-minus cork-screw pattern in Figure 3.7C. This back-and-forth shifting of the electric field charge is an electric vibration, and it is similar to what happens around a wire conducting alternating current (AC), like the alternating current in household wiring. The technical terms for electric vibration in neuroscience and physics are *oscillation* and *resonance*. In this book the term *electric vibration* will often be used because back-and-forth activity seems more easily visualized than alternating electric charge.

The electric vibration of the apical dendrite fiber bears some similarity to the mechanical vibration of the wire of a guitar or a violin. The main difference between them, of course, is that electric vibration is a plus-to-minus shift of an electric charge (which does not require physical movement), while the mechanical vibration is a back-and-forth movement of physical material of an object.

Electric vibrations of an apical dendrite are produced by surges of current being fed into it at the top as shown in Figure 3.7. A picture of electric surges in an apical dendrite is very different than a picture of electric pulses in an axon. A train of surges produces a smooth wave shape like the one shown by the corkscrew in Figure 3.7, while a train of spikes resembles the row of teeth on the shaft of a comb (see Figure 2.6, bottom). Also, spikes and surges move along a neural fiber in very different ways. A surge of electric charges passes smoothly along the inside of the fiber, but a spike jumps along its fiber. A neural fiber reacts somewhat passively to the slight increase in voltage intensity of a surge of current, but when a spike occurs, the neural fiber responds actively, by suddenly thrusting charged particles out of the neuron. Also, a surge of current has a lower voltage intensity than the voltage necessary to produce a spike. Hence, surges of electric current usually move down the apical dendrite without producing spikes.

The title of this chapter is a question: "Is Mental Life More Than Processing Information?" The answer of this book is a resounding "yes," and Figure 3.7 shows what that "more" involves. It consists of electric vibrations (electric resonating) of apical dendrites. The resonating apical dendrites in their loop circuits join the processing of electric pulses in network circuits to produce our mental life.

The takeaway message from this chapter is that apical dendrites do not have as their main function the moving of pulses of information from one place to another place like other neural fibers do. Instead, the vibrations of apical dendrites stay where they are and continue to vibrate for a period of time. The next chapter describes the other things that apical dendrites do to make possible our daily mental life.

This chapter reviewed the apical dendrite of the pyramidal neuron, including its neural structure and its neural workings. The conclusion is that the main function of the apical dendrite is not to move pulse information from one place to another place like the moving of electric spikes. Instead, the apical dendrite vibrates electrically to the pulses delivered to it. This vibration does not move along a fiber that is connected to another neuron but instead stays in one place within its loop circuit and continues to vibrate for a while. For these reasons, the vibrating apical dendrite can be described as a *state* of mental activity, instead of as one event acting on another event in the brain, like a spike produces another spike on an axon.

A glance at the meshwork of the neural network in Figure 3.4 shows spikes that are moving from one place to another, and the pathways of these spikes branch to make more and more pathways for the electric pulses as they move deeper into the brain. So, according to this picture, wires in computers and fibers in the brain both carry electric pulses from one location to another. In other words, both computers and brains process and move information.

The computer metaphor works for the brain because both computers and brains contain circuits whose wiring patterns have a network structure. A network circuit makes it possible for "everything to be connected to everything," which is particularly effective for storing information about different kinds of things. In contrast, circuits that have wiring patterns like separated loop circuits produce situations where "you can't get there from here," which prevent some parts of a wiring system from communicating with each other. This difference in wiring patterns between network circuitry and loop circuitry is a hardware feature that sets apart computer activity from apical dendrite activity. In a network circuit, spikes are sent from one location to another to communicate information; in loop circuits spikes stay in their loop circuit and cause the apical dendrite to vibrate (resonate) electrically.

Chapter 4

How the Vibrating Apical Dendrite Works

When Louis Armstrong, the famous jazz trumpeter, was asked to define jazz he replied, "If you have to ask what jazz is, you'll never know." Another musician said, "You don't define jazz, you dig it." Everyone knows that feelings cannot be defined. But, perhaps the words "dig it" could call up some vibrating apical dendrites and give you the feeling of jazz, or the feeling of returning to your first home, or the feeling of seeing a mountain. When you "dig" something, you are using a part of the brain where words never go.

Many diagrams in this book offer visual images of what the apical dendrite is doing while we experience a feeling, and also while we see a painting or hear music. The active apical dendrite can be imagined as an electric vibration, during which the dendrite fiber shifts its electric charges back and forth from positive to negative again and again. Usually, these electrical vibrations are very rapid.

For many people, the image of a vibrating string is familiar, but they have no visual image of a vibrating electric charge. Figure 4.1 shows the physical structure of the apical dendrite and its activity. For most of us, the word vibration calls up an image of a string stretched

The Apical Dendrite in a Loop Circuit

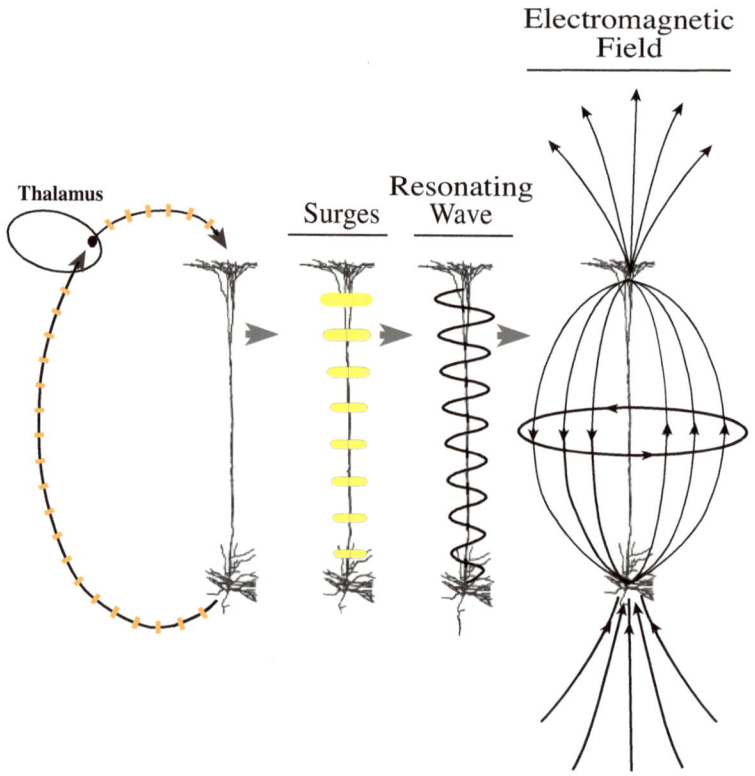

Figure 4.1

between two fixed points that rapidly moves up and down. When you pull the string with your finger and suddenly let it go sometimes you can actually see the hills and valleys of the vibration. This image of a rapidly moving string could be used to compare electric vibrating with the movement of surges along a wire or a fiber. A misleading feature of this image is that it is a mechanical image, an image of a physical object that is moving up and down or side-to-side, whereas an electric vibration involves changing electric charges on parts of that object.

When we grasp a wire that is carrying a mild electric charge the changes from positive to negative charge are transmitted to our skin. But the feeling of the electric vibration is different than feeling the slow vibration of a guitar string on your finger tip. A charged electric wire may even make your hand and arm jump if the electric charges penetrate to muscles. In short, while a mechanical vibration involves a change in location of something, an electric vibration involves a change in the electric charge of something. Resonating, in its technical sense, is simply another word for vibrating, and is also used in daily conversation when someone else has experienced an emotion or an idea that you have had. Saying that you resonate with them is the same as saying that you vibe with them, which means that you vibrate with them.

The Unseen Light Inside the Brain

When the apical dendrite vibrates electrically, it radiates electromagnetic waves outward. Figure 4.1 shows this radiation pattern by the diagram on the right end of the drawings. The downward movement of current surges produces an electric vibration of the apical dendrite, which produces the wave pattern of electromagnetic radiation. The direction of electric radiation is the vertical direction because the apical dendrite is oriented in that direction. The magnetic part of the radiation, represented by the circular field at the center of the diagram, is oriented in the horizontal direction.

The light waves produced by the apical dendrite are not seen by us because they are located in an invisible part of the range (spectrum) of electromagnetic radiation, as shown in Figure 4.2. The label for the visible part of the spectrum is located under the rainbow colors of the spectrum. Also labeled are invisible parts of the spectrum that produce X-rays, radio waves, and resonance waves of apical dendrites.

At the top of Figure 4.2 is a horizontal wave that is changing its frequency from slow to fast in the left-to-right direction. The frequency of a wave is based on counting the number of repetitions (cycles) of the motion of the wave in a second of time, for example it counts the number of wave peaks in a second. The magnitude (amplitude) of the apical dendrite wave is indicated by how far its peaks diverge from its center. The magnitude of the apical dendrite wave is directly proportional to the length of the apical dendrite.

Apical dendrites can resonate only at frequencies between zero and 1,000 cycles per second, because that is the range of pulse frequencies for the pulse inputs to the apical dendrite. This range puts the apical dendrite's range of frequencies at the low end of the electromagnetic spectrum shown in Figure 4.2, well away from the range of visible light. But the apical dendrite still gives off light because it is an electromagnetic wave. Imagine that at any moment of our waking life, millions of apical dendrites are lighting up our brain with this unseen, dark light.

Evidence from EEG Recordings that Apical Dendrites Vibrate Electrically

The existence of brain waves is a common fact and most people have heard of the electroencephalograph (EEG). This is a device that records brain waves by placing small button-like discs on the head, as shown in Figure 4.3. Some of the kinds of brain waves revealed by EEG recordings are shown in Figure 4.4. Each of the recordings was made while the person was observed to be in a particular mental state,

The Electromagnetic Wave Spectrum

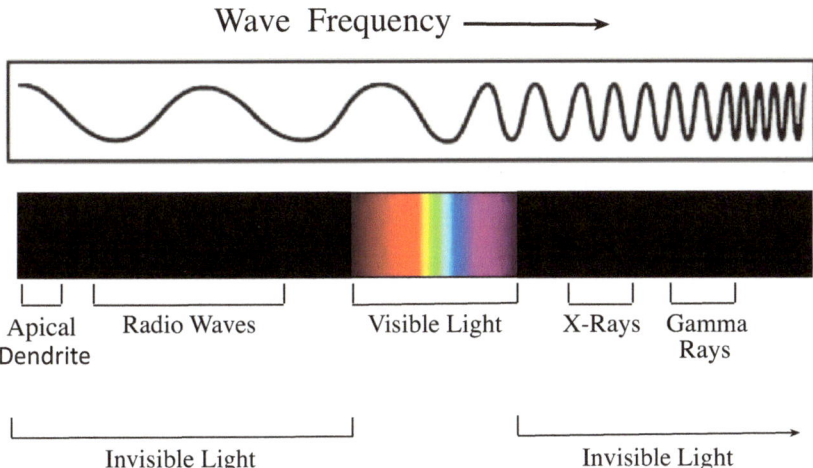

Figure 4.2

from excitement for the top recording to coma for the bottom recording. The excited wave pattern of the top recording is produced by individuals while they are engaged in everyday activities, such as talking on the phone or working at the computer. The relaxed wave pattern is found when a person is calm and stares mindlessly at the wall or out the window. The wave patterns observed during other daily activities tend to fall somewhere between the excited pattern and the relaxed pattern.

The frequency range of the waves that make up the excitement pattern starts at about 30 cycles per second and can reach as high as 120 cycles per second, all labeled gamma waves. The frequency range of waves of the relaxed pattern are 8 to 12 cycles per second; these waves are labeled alpha waves. A glance at the two patterns shows the complexity of the gamma waves during a state of excitement and the simplicity of the alpha waves. The excitement waves show a mixture of many different frequencies. This seems to indicate that the many different regions of the cortex are doing different things when you are excited, while the alpha wave seems to be dominated by one frequency, which seems to indicate that different regions of the cortex are doing the same thing when you are relaxed.

The main source of these EEG waves is the apical dendrite. The wave from one apical dendrite is not strong enough to be recorded at the scalp, especially if the wave must travel through a lot of cortical tissue to reach a particular recording pad at the scalp. It takes thousands of apical dendrites resonating at the same frequency to produce a clear wave recording at the scalp. The EEG records the electric part of electromagnetic waves. In Figure 4.1, the drawing of the electromagnetic field shows the magnetic part of the electromagnetic field as a circular shape. The magnetic field sends its waves outward in the horizontal direction, and these magnetic waves are relatively undisturbed when traveling through brain tissue while electric waves undergo significant disturbance. The device that records these waves is called the

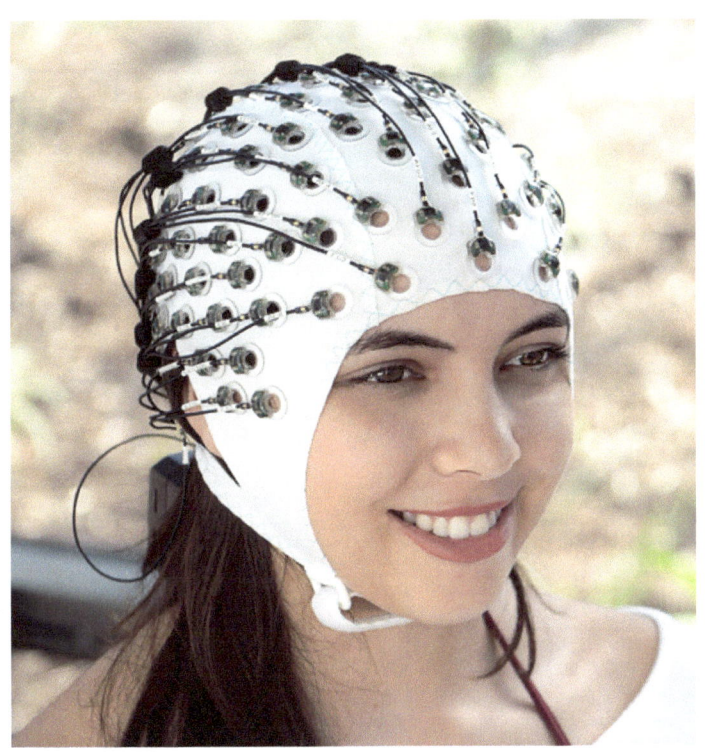

Figure 4.3

Types of Brain Waves (EEGs)

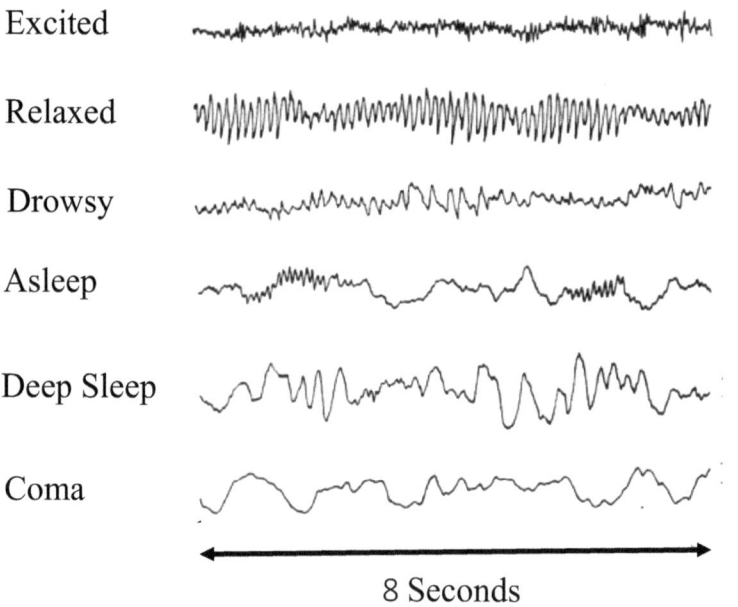

Excited

Relaxed

Drowsy

Asleep

Deep Sleep

Coma

8 Seconds

Figure 4.4

magneto-encephalograph (MEG), and it is used to pinpoint the brain location of the apical dendrites that are beaming out electric waves as well as magnetic waves.

The EEG measurement has provided ample evidence of the resonating of the apical dendrites in the cortex, activity that is always going on during waking and sleeping. Computers, which do not contain apical dendrites, do not show this kind of electric wave activity arising from their network grid because they do not contain clusters of loop circuits. The evolutionary appearance in the mammalian brain of large numbers of apical dendrites marks the beginning of the influence of the apical dendrite loop circuit on the workings of the brain. The degree of this influence increased considerably as the length of the apical dendrite increased from the mouse to the human.

This chapter began with the question of how you define jazz, and answered that you don't define jazz, you "dig" it. That is, when you hear jazz you get a certain kind of feeling. For many thoughtful readers, the words *dig* and *feeling* do not really help them understand why jazz can't be defined, mainly because the reader is left up in the air about what dig and feeling themselves mean. It seems that in our search for understanding words like jazz, feelings, good, evil, and love, we always seem to find ourselves using more words to define words. Can we escape from this box of words by looking into the brain to see what it is doing when we use words? Could loop circuits offer us a new way to understand what the brain is doing when we encounter undefinable words like *dig* and *feeling*?

Chapter 5

The Two Neural Systems of Our Mental Life: A Brief Summary

This chapter takes the main points of the previous chapters and tries to put them together in one picture so that we can see how the network and loop circuits are both active while we perform the many familiar tasks of everyday life. But before doing this, it will help to draw the resonating apical dendrite in another way, a way that emphasizes its electrical features. The new drawing of the apical dendrite is based on a method that EEG researchers have used for many years to find the locations in the brain of the EGG electric waves that they record[1].

Locating a Cluster of Apical Dendrites in the Brain
As noted earlier, the EEG takes its recordings from many locations around the skull surface. A single cluster of apical dendrites located anywhere in the cortex will beam its electric waves at the same time to the EEG pads at these different locations. For example, one pad may be located at the top of the head, one above and behind the left ear, and another above and in front of the right ear. These three points form triangles with the apical dendrite cluster in three dimensions and makes

it possible to work backwards to pinpoint the location of that cluster of apical dendrites in the 3-D space of the cortex.

The cluster of apical dendrites that beams the electric waves outward can be represented as a cylinder that has opposite charges at each end and it is called a *dipole*. As the name suggests, a dipole is a pair of equal and oppositely charged electric poles or two separated magnetic poles. A bar magnet is an example of a magnetic dipole and an apical dendrite is an example of an electric dipole. The electric dipole of the cluster is made up of the dipoles of each apical dendrite contained in the cluster. Figure 5.1 shows the electric dipole made by a single apical dendrite of a pyramidal neuron. (Note the similarities of the drawings of Figure 5.1 to the drawings in Figures 3.7 and 4.1). The plus and minus charges can be seen at the ends of the electric dipole.

The charges reverse their two locations as a surge of charges (with a gap between charges) moves down the apical dendrite. The surges in the apical dendrite begin at the top and when a surge of current enters the apical dendrite, the charges at the ends of the apical dendrite take on their positive or negative signs. When a gap between charges appears the charges reverse their signs and when a another surge appears the charges reverse signs again. Every reverse of charge makes the electromagnetic field, shown Figure 4.1, flip the direction that it sends out its electric radiation by 180 degrees. In this way, the electric wave sent from the apical dendrite to the three electrode pads on the skull produces the peaks (positive charge) and valleys (negative charge) in EEG recordings.

Locations of Major Cognitive Functions in the Brain

Chapter 3 described the role of the thalamus in sending neural pulses from the senses to the cortex, which will help understand the way the pyramidal neuron and its apical dendrite operate within the context of the whole brain. Figure 5.2 shows a cutaway view of the brain, which reveals the white-colored axons in the interior of the brain and a cut-

The Electric Dipole

Resonating
Dendrite

Dipole

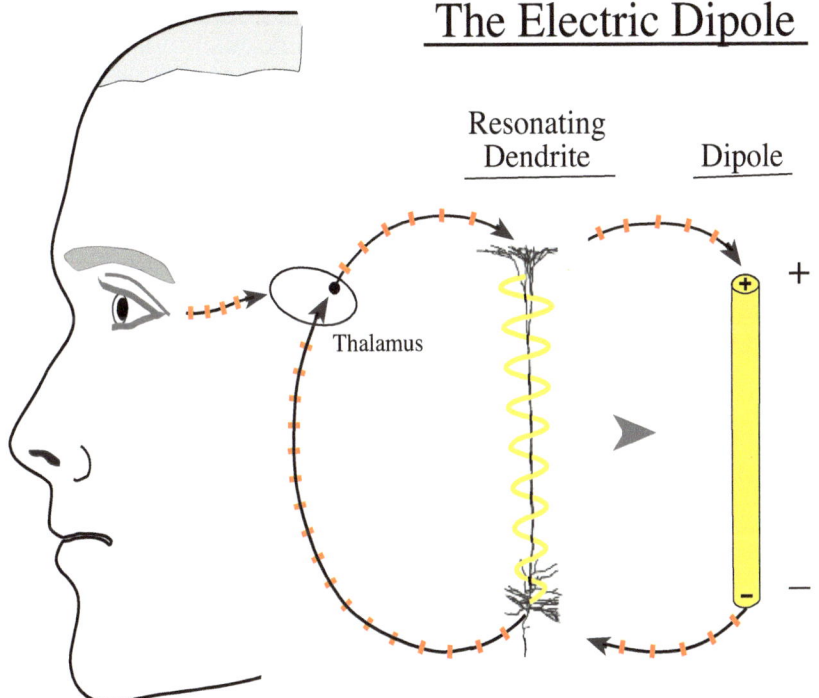

Thalamus

+

−

Figure 5.1

away view of the large sheet of networks (coded blue) that surrounds the large white interior of the brain.

This drawing shows both the loops (black ovals) and the network grid (blue ribbon) activity in a whole-brain diagram as a person is looking at something. Since this picture is a cutaway view of the left side of the brain when it is sliced vertically, the grid of the network system is shown as a thin band that is located near the outer surface of the cortex. So, this band of the network grid shows only the thickness of the large grid that spreads over the left side of the brain (see Figure 2.4).

Figure 5.2 shows that electric pulses from the eye first contact the thalamus, where they cause pulses to be sent directly to the network system (blue ribbon) in the part of the brain where visual features of objects and scenes are registered. It also shows that the thalamus is activating the network system of neurons indirectly by means of a loop circuit (colored black). The loop structure determines that once pulses enter the loop circuit the pulses keep moving, so that the pulse inputs from the eye do not stop but instead continue to refresh the objects or scenes registered in the brain. In this manner we can continue to see a person's face via the loop circuit while we use network circuits to choose the words we want to say to the person. In contrast, inside the computer-like network pulses cease once the series of input pulses is processed and the outputs sent to another part of the network.

The loop circuit contains only two neurons (the "sending" neuron from the thalamus to a dipole in the cortex and the "sending back" neuron from the cortex to the thalamus), which is much simpler than a typical circuit of the computer-like network in the brain. In a network, pathways resemble highways on a map, highways that wander far away from their original beginnings and often branch into more pathways. In a loop circuit, the pathway resembles the map of a simple racetrack that circles back on itself (see Figure 3.4).

The appearance of axon connections in the network system are shown by the blue lines in Figure 5.3. The shortest axons are located

From the Eye to the Network
And Loop Circuits

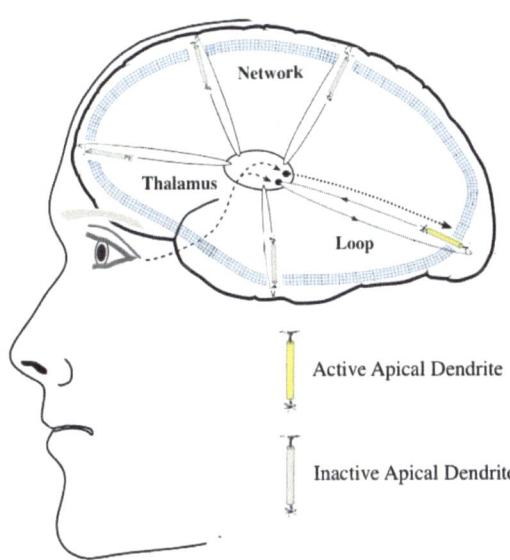

Figure 5.2

in the broad, relatively thin cortical sheet shown as a blue ribbon that covers the surface of the brain. Longer axons connect neighboring cortical areas to each other, shown as groups of small crescent-shaped connections. The longest axons cross the cortex in groups and connect with cortical areas that are located far from their sources. It should be observed in Figure 5.3 that these long axons (coded blue) are part of the network system and do not engage the thalamus.

When visual activity is first registered in the cortex (see Figure 5.2) it is sent to higher levels in the brain where it can be processed in different ways, as illustrated in Figure 5.4. The first stage of visual processing, located in the lower right corner of the drawing, is directly connected (via a neuron in the thalamus) to some of the other loops, for example, to the "where" and "what" loops (the connection between loops is not shown here, but can be seen by looking ahead to Figure 8.4). The connection between loops is made in the thalamus where the cortex-to-thalamus axon of one loop branches to contact the thalamic neuron of another loop.

In Figure 5.4 the psychological activity in the network neurons at the end of each loop is indicated by the label placed outside the surface of the brain. These particular locations become active when a person looks out the window and sees something. If the person hears something, the labels would change their locations, much more in the back part of the brain which specializes in sensory processing, than in the front part of the brain which specializes in the processing of actions to sensory inputs (for example, we use the same action of pointing to an object whether it is seen or heard).

For simplicity, Figure 5.4 omits showing an apical dendrite that represents clusters of cortical thalamic loops in the motor area, which is located at the top of the cortex. The circuitry in the motor response area is more complicated than other areas marked with a cluster of yellow apical dendrites[2]. Apparently, the sustaining of a command to a muscle group in the body involves thalamus-to-cortex circuitry that

Network Circuits Include Long Axons that Cross the Cortex and Short Axons Within The Grid Near the Surface of the Cortcx

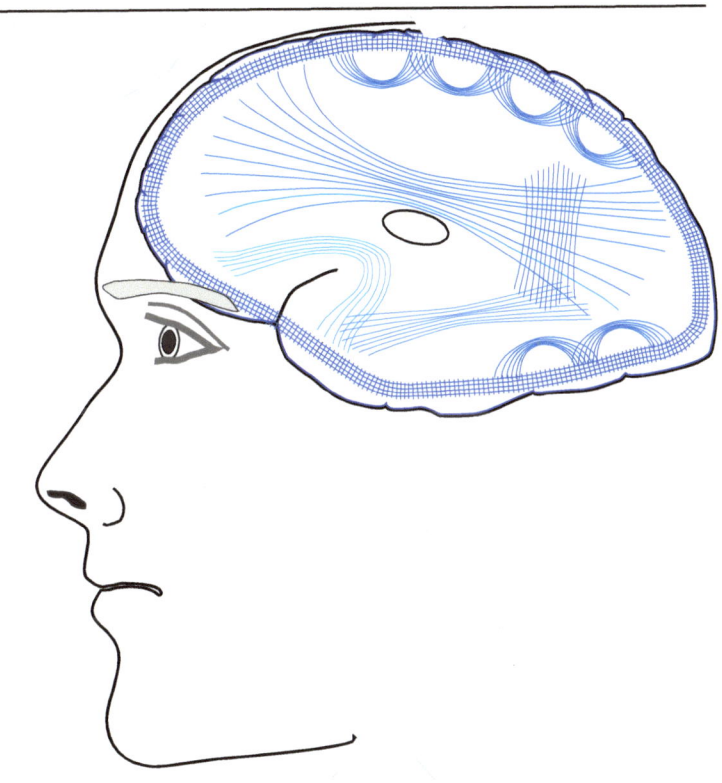

Figure 5.3

Loop Circuits Connect the Thalamus to Apical Dendrite Clusters that Serve Specific Psychological Functions

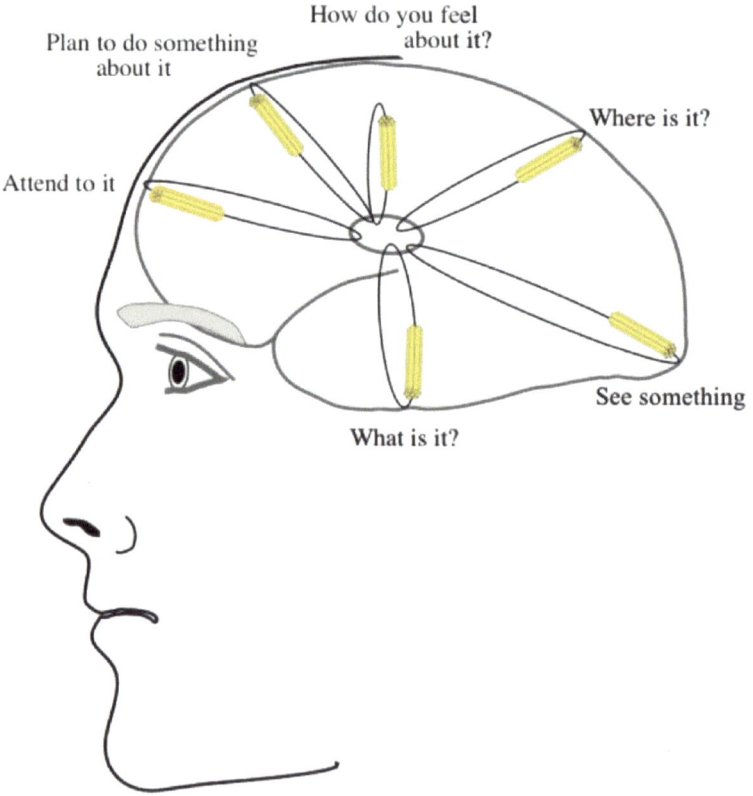

Figure 5.4

produce inhibitory actions as well as excitatory actions. Therefore, activation of the motor area by the apical dendrite should consist of two loops, one that excites motor neurons, and another that leads to the inhibiting of nearby motor neurons that serve similar responses. This complication is not surprising, since the execution of a response usually must also block the unwanted actions of other responses. Commanding a particular finger to move during playing a musical scale requires precise inhibition of other fingers. Alcohol inhibits the inhibitory neurons, and violinists and pianists know very well that drinking a glass of wine before playing a piece at a fast tempo risks blurring fast runs of notes.

This chapter was concerned with an overall view of the way the loop and network systems are both active while an individual is awake and engaged in daily activities. A detailed description of how a loop circuit influences the input-output activity of a network circuit will be presented in Chapter 10. The next chapter will examine the simple ways that the apical dendrite makes it possible to sustain and intensify attention.

Chapter 6

The Role of the Apical Dendrite in Attention

While reading a book or an article, did you ever use a highlighter to draw attention to a word or group of words? Some readers find themselves covering whole pages with their highlighter, and as a result, nothing remains to draw attention to particular words that have just been read. But, perhaps the movement of the pen over the words as they are read helps to concentrate attention on them while the eye moves over them. In other words, for some readers, the movement of the highlighter pen may act like an extension of their attention during reading.

One of the unanticipated discoveries that emerged in the development of the theory of the vibrating apical dendrite is a new way of describing how the brain produces attention, in particular the way that attention can be sustained and intensified. One way that the intensity of attention can be changed is by changing the length of the apical dendrite. Figure 3.2 shows that the length of the apical dendrite varies greatly among species of mammals. This has important implications for generalizing results of an attention experiment from one species to another. For example, selective attention circuits that contain apical dendrites in pyramidal neurons will be much weaker in mice than in humans.

Another way that the intensity of attention is changed is by firing several spikes close together in what is called a burst[1]. The right side of Figure 6.1 shows examples of burst firing of spike pulses, and the left side of Figure 6.1 shows the steady single-spike pulses of regular firing.

The theory of loop circuits in this book proposes that attention can increase the intensity of the loop circuit activity by shifting from regular firing of single spikes to the burst firing of spikes. This often happens when we are looking at something and then adjust our attention to a higher level. Waiting for a red traffic light to turn green seems to involve little or no attention. But if the intention is to make a fast start, attention is raised in anticipation of the moment that the light changes from red to green. In a similar manner, when you hear footsteps in the hallway outside your door, you not only move your attention to the door (in anticipation of the sound of a knock), but if the sound of the footsteps stops outside your door the intensity of your attention may suddenly increase to its peak level.

Anticipating the moment an upcoming event will occur usually increases the number of pulses in the bursts that move within the relevant loop circuits. It turns out that a neural burst can contain any number of spikes up to about seven, which can be observed by counting the spikes crowded into one of the four bursts shown on the right side of Figure 6.1.

Henceforth, in the figures of this book it will be helpful to represent the low and high levels of attention by changing the color of the yellow resonating neuron to orange for low attention or to red for high attention. Figure 6.2 shows these three color codes in the bottom row of the drawing; in the top row, this figure shows corresponding bursts of one, two, or four pulses in the loop circuits; and in the central row the waves show greater intensities by their higher peaks and deeper valleys. Figure 6.3 shows a cat that is staring at something with very intense attention, and we can easily imagine the face of a person showing the same intensity when attending strongly to an automobile chase scene on television.

Rhythmic Single Pulses   Rhythmic Bursts

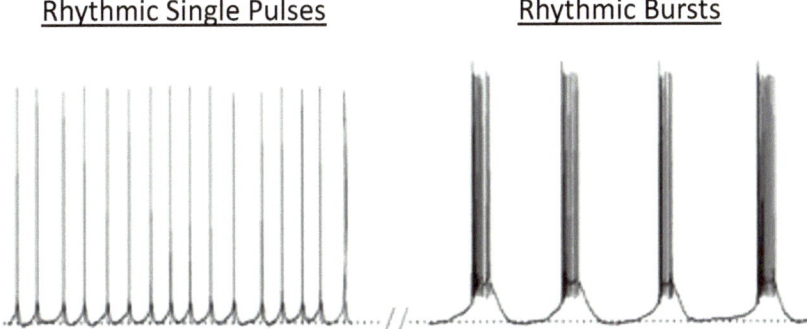

Figure 6.1

Levels of Attention and Color Codes

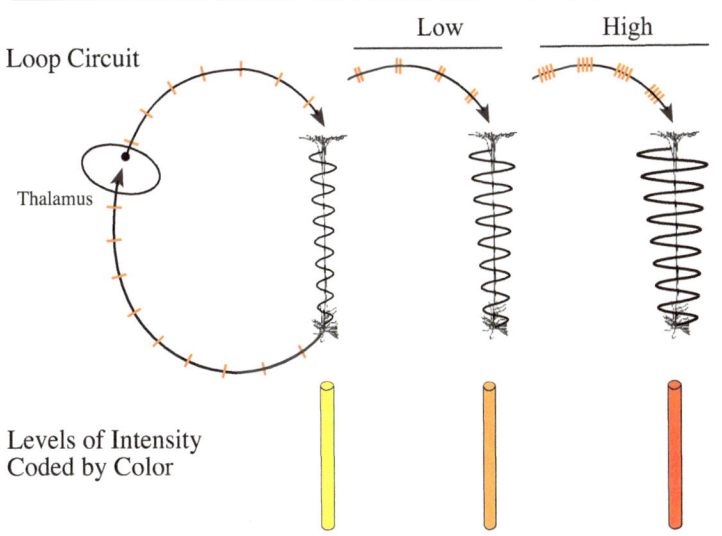

Figure 6.2

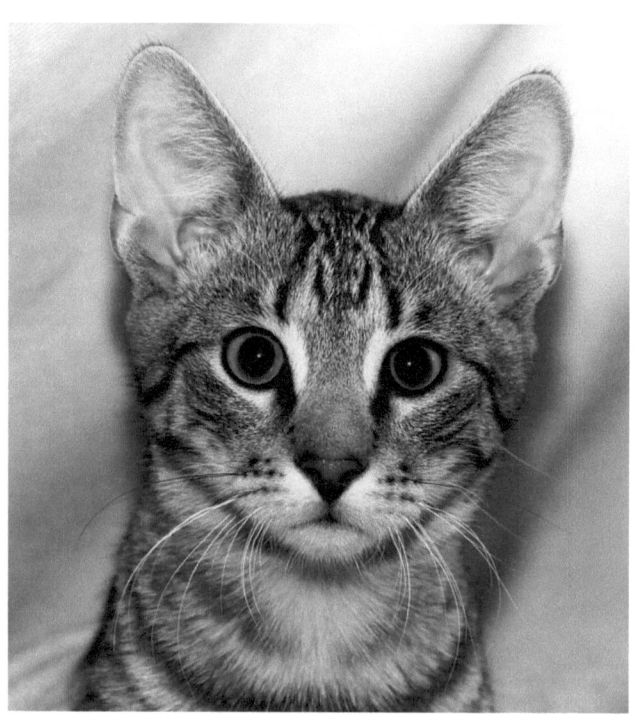

Figure 6.3

The levels of attentional intensity made possible by the burst firing of neurons has implications for the role of the arts in our lives. The English poet and critic, T. E. Hulme, who lived at the beginning of the 20th century, believed that most people do not perceive things vividly and that they can only be made to do so by the artist. He wrote:

> *In ordinary life, I realize a given object, say,*
> *with the given intensity two. An artist*
> *realizes this with the intensity four, and by*
> *his manner of emphasizing it makes me*
> *realize it with the same intensity.* [2]

How does the brain intensify the images it perceives using attention? The answer is by a loop ciruit that contains the thalamus.

Evidence that the Thalamus is Involved in Attention

A key assumption of the loop theory is that the attention-producing apical dendrite is connected to the thalamus. Neuroscientists had suspected for some time that the thalamus is involved in attention, but in the 1980's and 1990's, experiments began to establish the direct involvement of the thalamus during the performance of attention-demanding tasks[3,4]. One of these experiments, reported in 1990, was carried out by Monte Buchsbaum and myself at the University of California, Irvine[5]. In this experiment, brain scans were carried out immediately following each of two tasks: a task that required a high level of attention and a task that required a very low-level of attention. The high-attention task was similar to identifying a face at the center of a photograph of a group of faces, but instead of faces, the objects to be identified were letters that were similar to each other. In the low-attention task, the target letter was much larger and was displayed alone. The brain scans showed higher activity in the back part of the thalamus when the target letter was surrounded by other letters than when it was large and displayed alone.

On the left side of Figure 6.4 is a magnetic resonance image (MRI) from one of the participants in the 1990 experiment. This photograph shows a horizontal slice that extends from the forehead region to the back of the head. On the right side of Figure 6.4 is a drawing that shows the same outline of the brain slice in the photograph and contains the smaller outlines of the thalamus and some the parts of the thalamus. This figure shows the outlines of the back part of the thalamus and the middle top of the thalamus, which are the largest and second largest parts (nuclei), respectively, of the thalamus. The back region of the thalamus is named the *pulvinar* (pulvinar means "pillow" in Latin and is assumed to be the largest object in the thalamic bed). The pulvinar is the part of the thalamus that is of special interest in the 1990 experiment because, as mentioned earlier, it has direct connections to the area of the cortex that specializes in processing visual objects, including letters. The middle top area of the thalamus has direct connections to the attention control area and to the feelings area of the insula (a thumb-sized cortical area located slightly above and in front of the ear). It is well known that loop circuits connect most areas of the cortex to the thalamus, and that these circuits can synchronize activity between the thalamus and these areas of the cortex[6].

This experiment was later repeated in a 2006 study[7] that used the same letter-identification displays of the 1990 study. The results of the 2006 experiment confirmed the main results of the 1990 experiment by showing that the back part (pulvinar nucleus) of the thalamus was more active in the high-attention task than in the low attention task. The 2006 experiment, which used more advanced scanning technology than was available for the 1990 experiment, provided evidence that other locations within the thalamus are involved in attention (see Figure 6.4, right side). The scans revealed the participation of the middle top part (mediodorsal nucleus) of the thalamus, which is connected to the frontal cortical area, which supports the control of attention, as well as to the insula area which supports subjective feelings.

The Thalamus: One in Each Hemisphere

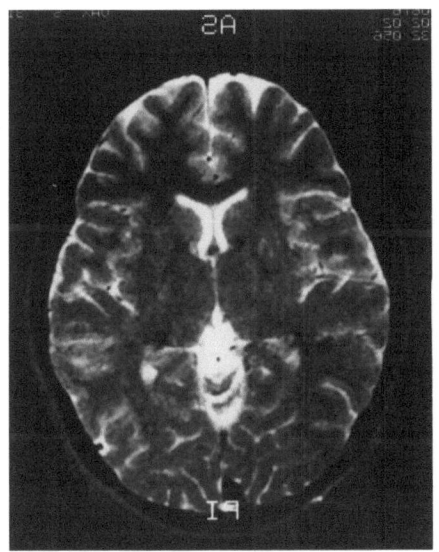 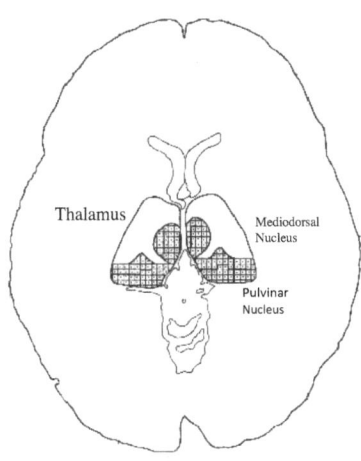

Figure 6.4

Choosing What to Attend To

The scene inside a room or outside through a window typically contains many objects, and one particular object usually commands our attention for a few seconds or minutes. Meanwhile the person standing next to you may be attending to another object. What holds our attention is usually a matter of personal choice.

The choosing of what to attend to during the passing moments of daily living can be represented by choosing a channel on television or choosing a station of a radio. Figure 6.5 shows a dial on the left side of the figure that chooses the frequency of a TV channel or radio station on the right side of the figure. The broadcasting stations are indicated by towers that have an antenna at the top that sends out electric signals carried on a wave that is set at the frequency shown by the wave underneath the towers.

A television or radio is connected to an antenna that receives the signals sent out from all of the four broadcasting stations, but in order to show and/or hear what a particular station is sending out, there must be a way to select radio signals only from that station. Since a station is identified by the frequency of the signals it beams, the television receiver needs only to select that frequency among all the frequencies that its antenna is receiving. The choice of a broadcasting station is made by turning the dial to the station that currently has the most appealing program. The same kind of diagram shown in Figure 6.5 can be transferred to the brain, and it is shown in Figure 6.6. Here, each broadcasting station is replaced by a cluster of apical dendrites in which all resonate at the same frequency. Clusters of apical dendrites resonate to the appearance of a visual object, the location of that object, a sound, or to bodily inputs that produce feelings (see Figure 5.4). On the left side of Figure 6.6 is the "dial" in the frontal area of the brain that chooses which of these clusters of apical dendrites will dominate our experience at that moment.

The decision to shift the firing level of an apical dendrite cluster is also carried out in the frontal area of the brain, which is located on the

Choosing Which Radio
Station to Dial Up

Tuning to a Station Frequency	Sources of a Radio Frequency Signal

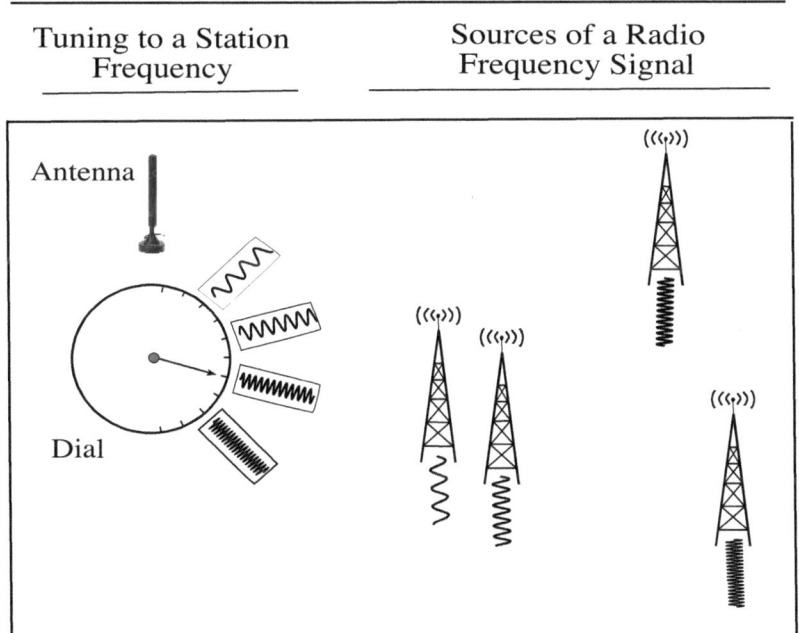

Figure 6.5

Choosing What To Attend To

Attentional Choices	Major Inputs to the Brain

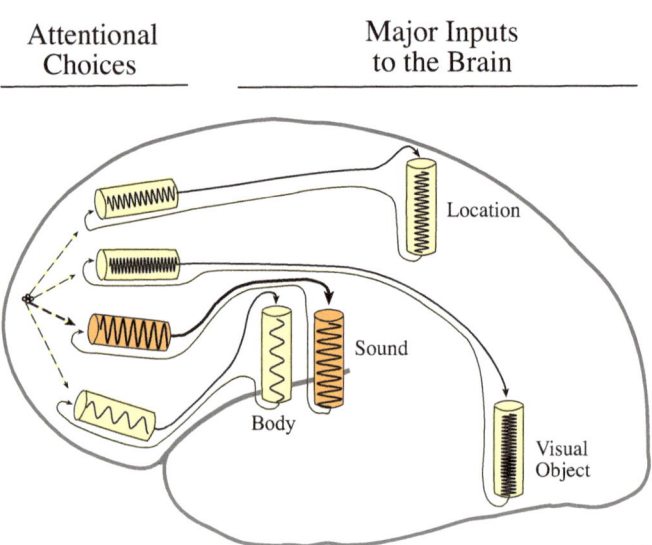

Figure 6.6

left side of Figure 6.6. This brain region contains the circuits that control attention, and clusters of apical dendrites in four loop circuits are drawn here as choice alternatives. The input that activates each cluster is indicated by a line that comes from the neuron "dial" on the left of the clusters.

When pulses from the neuron "dial" shift the firing level from single-spikes to bursts of spikes in specific circuits of apical dendrites in the control area, a train of bursts is sent by way of the thalamus, via loop circuits, to the apical dendrite cluster in one of the regions of the brain shown on the right side of Figure 6.6. In this way, the neurons of the brain connect the voluntary choice of what you want to attend to its representation in the brain. For example, when you are watching a singer on television you can attend to the visual impression of the singer, the music she is singing, or to the feelings that you get while you hear the music.

Another look at the attention region on the left side of Figure 6.6 raises the question of what controls the "dial" neuron so that it sends burst pulses to what you want to attend to. Currently it is not known exactly how this voluntary choice is made, but we know that circuits in this frontal region of the cortex are active while attending to something, and we know that this activity is influenced by the motivational appeal of the attended object or of the feelings that go with that object.

A frequent question that is raised about the control of attention is, "If attention intensifies the activity of apical dendrites, why doesn't the subjective appearance of the object that we are attending to become more intense also? For example, when we attend to a word of text or to a face in a crowd, why doesn't the appearance of the word or face become brighter? The answer is that axons from the frontal area of attention control do not directly contact neurons in the primary visual cortex, but only indirectly by way of synapses in higher areas of visual processing, and this indirect route to the primary visual area may not engage the loop circuits of vision and their pyramidal neurons in the manner that the direct route from the eye does. This indirect way of connecting the voluntary areas of attention control to the primary visual areas of experiencing objects seems to be a good thing because it prevents the frontal area from changing the brain's registration of objects that are received from the eyes, which, like wearing distorting lenses, could endanger our life in risky situations, such as crossing a street in a busy city.

Bundles and Clusters of Apical Dendrites

In the chapters that follow, the kinds of things that the apical dendrite can do in our mental life will sometimes involve groups of apical dendrites instead of a single apical dendrite. For present purposes groupings of seven apical dendrites represent a *bundle*, and any grouping of bundles larger than two will represent a *cluster*. A bundle and a cluster of resonating apical dendrites are shown in Figure 6.7, along with a single apical dendrite, and to the left of these displays is the pyramidal neuron with a resonating wave moving down the apical dendrite. The color of the apical dendrites is yellow to represent an active state that is less intense than a state of attention.

A cluster of apical dendrites is usually surrounded by apical dendrites that have never been active, particularly for individuals who have had little exposure to the objects represented by the apical dendrites. Figure 6.8 shows a cutaway drawing of a cluster of bundles of active apical dendrites surrounded by bundles of inactive apical dendrites. The active apical dendrites are colored yellow, and the inactive apical dendrites are colored grey. The bundle of active apical dendrites could represent a visual scene being registered in the brain but not attended, for example, looking out of the window of an airplane while concentrating on the music in your earphones.

When attention is shifted from the music to an object outside the window of the airplane, as for example to another airplane, the cluster of apical dendrites representing the sight of that airplane will be shifted

Loop Circuits

Active Apical Dendrite: Alone, in a Bundle, and in a Cluster of Bundles

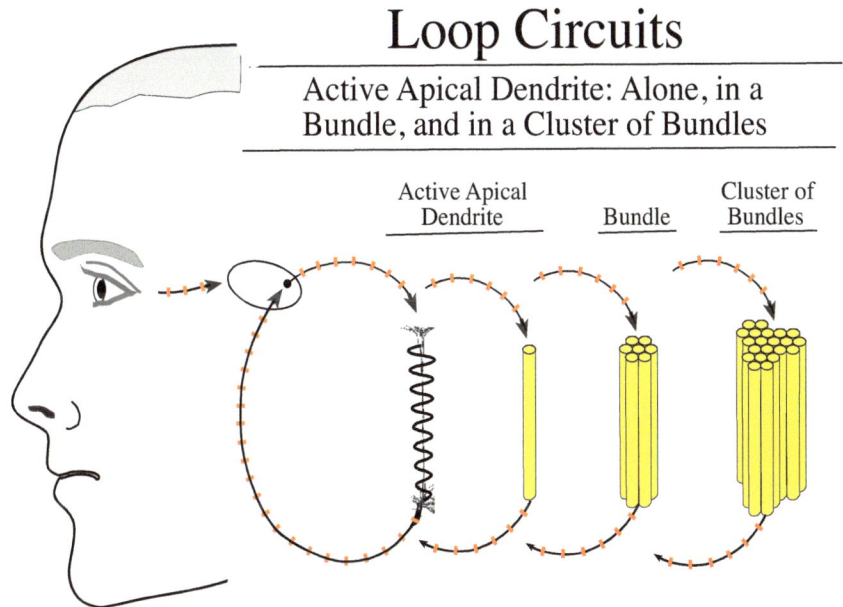

Figure 6.7

Activated Apical Dendrites Nested Inside of Unactivated Apical Dendrites

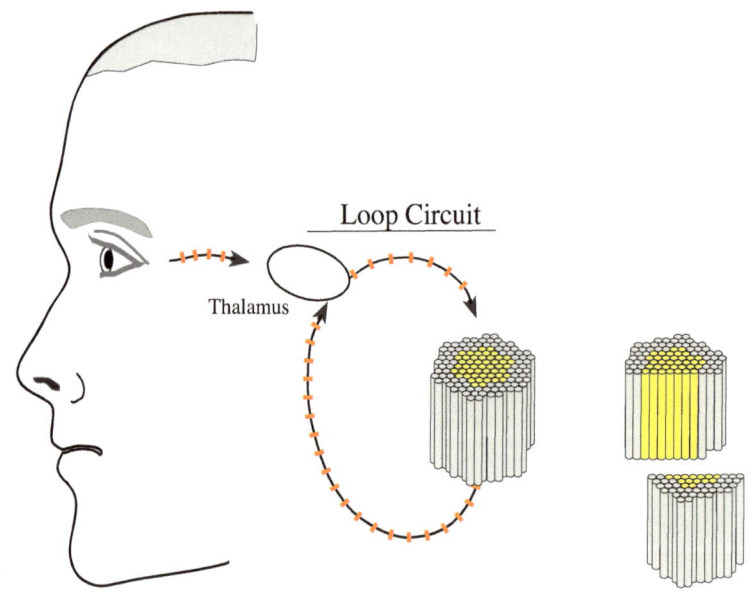

Figure 6.8

from unattended to a low level of attention. If there is something unusual or threatening about the movements of the other airplane, then the intensity of attention will shift to a higher level. The color codes for clusters having these levels of activity are shown in Figure 6.9.

Attending to an object involves more than raising the intensity of clusters of apical dendrites that represent that object. Pyramidal neurons in the attended cluster also send out pulses that inhibit the pyramidal neurons located in the lateral cortical neighborhood that represent objects that are similar to the attended object. However, axon outputs of pyramidal neurons do not themselves inhibit other neurons, they only excite them. The way that nearby pyramidal neurons are inhibited is by exciting the small inhibitory neurons that surround them.

Typically, so many inhibitory axons contact the cell body of a pyramidal neuron that its cell body is virtually covered by inhibitory synapses. As a result, when these short inhibitory neurons are activated, they can easily diminish or even shut down the activity of the pyramidal neuron that they contact because it is the cell body itself that excites the single axon that transmits pulses to other neurons. Therefore, when each pyramidal neuron is activated it usually causes other pyramidal neurons in its vicinity to be inhibited.

This lateral inhibition between clusters of pyramidal neurons tells us how a magician uses misdirection to conceal how he or she pulls a rabbit out of a hat that had just been shown to be empty. While the empty top hat is sitting on the table, the magician makes a playing card disappear, and then reaches inside his jacket and, instead of pulling out the expected playing card, pulls out a large bouquet of flowers (a group of artificial flowers held together by a spring, that had been "loaded" into the jacket much earlier). At the moment that the audience is surprised by the appearance of the flowers now held high in one hand, the magician reaches under the table with the other hand and quickly transfers a small rabbit into the tall top hat. Then the magician introduces a new trick that ends with lifting the hat off the table and reaching inside it to pull out the live rabbit.

Apical Dendrite Clusters: Three Levels of Intensity

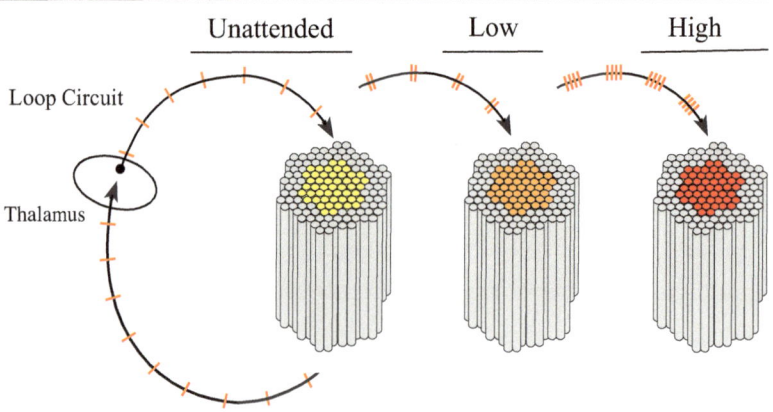

Figure 6.9

Even though the hat has been in plain sight when the rabbit was transferred to it, the attention of the audience was captured by the unexpected appearance of the large bouquet of flowers. The momentary attention to the flowers is typically very intense, owing to the surprise of suddenly seeing a large and colorful display of flowers. In the brains of the viewers, the cluster of pyramidal neurons corresponding to the location of the flowers is very strongly activated, which, in turn, strongly inhibits the activities of neighboring clusters that represent the locations of objects in the vicinity of the bouquet of flowers, including the location of the hat. In this way, the audience is made momentarily blind to anything happening except the experiencing of the flowers. Groups of axons that connect pyramidal neurons to the inhibitory neurons that surround neighboring pyramidal neurons can be observed in micro-photographs of the cortex[8].

Automatic Processing:
When Neural Processing Does Not Need Attention

Circuits that use single-pulse firing (yellow-coded circuits) also can produce responses automatically (i.e., without the burst firings involved in attention) when the stimulating object and the response are sufficiently familiar. For example, picking up the telephone while paying attention to getting dressed is possible because the ring of a telephone has been experienced often enough to build large clusters of activated apical dendrites and because the act of picking up a telephone also is supported by large clusters of apical dendrites (see Chapter 7). In addition, the connections between the two clusters have been strengthened by repeated experiencing of picking up a ringing phone.

The automatic processing of a task has been studied extensively, and in an early article (1974), Jay Samuels and I proposed a theory of automatic processing in reading[9]. When reading a line of text, mature readers do two things at the same time: they perceive words and comprehend them. Comprehension is usually the task that requires attention, especially when the material being read is new to the reader. Therefore, to become a good reader, the task of perceiving (often called decoding) the words must become automatic, so that full attention can be given to understanding what is being read.

These two tasks were believed to involve separate cognitive processes, which suggested that they could be investigated separately. With this two-task approach to the skill of reading, research on the teaching of reading in the schools could focus on one of these tasks at a time, either making word perception more automatic, or using attention more effectively in comprehension of strings of these words.

Another example of doing two tasks at the same time when one task is highly automatic is using the phone while driving. What makes this activity so tempting is that using the phone while driving involves many minutes in which little if any attention seems to be required for driving. However, what makes this activity dangerous is that in the moment when driving requires attention (a child at a crosswalk), something in the phone conversation may have already momentarily attracted the driver's attention. It is the infrequency of such moments that may tempt a person to pick up the phone while driving, but being recently reminded of the enormous cost of a tragic accident can resist that temptation.

According to the theory described in this book, the process of choosing what to attend to and for how long involves clusters of resonating apical dendrites. The movement of pulses around a resonating circuit is so rapid that it would seem difficult to pinpoint exactly the moment that a pulse sent from the loop circuit contacts a neuron in a decision circuit. So, one may wonder if the presence of resonating apical dendrites in the decision-making process makes the decision less predictable than processing in networks without apical dendrites. Does this element of unpredictably indicate that free will can operate in making a decision?

Is the Vibrating Apical Dendrite a Door to Free Will ?

In 1870, William James, the American philosopher and psychologist, described free will as "the sustaining of a thought because I choose to when I might have other thoughts." For James, this example of personal freedom in the act of thinking brought him out of a deep depression. He had been reading and thinking about how the mind works, and the available scientific evidence had convinced him that the mind's brain works by blind physical forces that act on each other, like a machine. Therefore, if you know the state of the brain at a particular time, you can predict exactly what the person will do next. For James, this was devastating because he strongly believed that the value of living is in the things you can accomplish as a person, and freedom in thinking was crucial to his belief in personal achievement.

Choosing to sustain a thought or even to sustain a perception "a bit longer," and then "just a bit longer," is very easy to demonstrate for oneself, for example, by trying to fix one's attention on a word of text. The visual sensation of the word does not stay still but wobbles ever so slightly. Similarly, allowing attention to a thought to continue or letting it shift to other thoughts is a choice between thoughts each of which wobbles uncontrollably. At the neural level, each thought is sustained in the mind by apical dendrite activity that involves small wobbles in timing and intensity of electric vibration. So, when choices are as close as the "sustain-or-shift-my-attention" choice, the exact moment of making the winning decision seems to be unpredictable.

In contrast, the process of comparing alternative decisions in computer circuits involves highly reliable wire-to-wire contacts, and there are no loop circuits with their wobbles in timing at the moment of sending an output signal. Today, it seems that the person-vs-machine crisis, described so persuasively by William James, has become the person-vs-the computer.

For James, his Dilemma of Determinism article[11] reconciled the difference between personal choice in the mind and the rigid cause-and-effect in the world outside the mind. He coined the terms *soft determinism* and *hard determinism* to distinguish between the two kinds of causality. The addition of elements of freedom and moral responsibility to personal choice makes it an example of soft determinism.

The contribution of resonating apical dendrites to the problem of freedom in thinking would be illuminated if a computer would be built that contains resonating loop circuits as well as networks. Would a machine version of the network-loop model produce EEGs like those of a human brain? Could the loop activity act as a clock that coordinates pulse timing in separate circuits? Could bursts of pulses in a circuit select one circuit over other active circuits for momentary processing? In any case, predicting the moment that a loop circuit impacts the activity in a network circuit is considerably more uncertain than predicting the moment that a network circuit impacts activity in another network circuit. The increase in temporal uncertainty seems to be a feature that is built in to the way the loop circuit works.

The two-systems view of this book described in Chapter 5 suggests an alternaitve theory of free will based on the distinction between thinking and feeling. To define free will involves network circuits that enable *thinking*, and to *feel* the action of choosing involves the apical dendrite in loop circuits. Consider a definition that asserts that free will is the apparent absence of a physical cause, something like the uncertainty principle of quantum physics. To approximate such a "causeless action" we usually use a haphazard device, like flipping a coin as a way of choosing an alternative. The problem with using a random method of choice in the brain is that the brain must obey that choice in a hard deterministic manner, and the particular choice actually made may be undesirable to the person. As a result, the *feeling* that accompanies the act of choosing may be perceived as having been coerced, which is the opposite of the feeling of having the freedom to choose.

On the other hand when you choose a particular flavor of ice cream because you like that flavor (and people who know you predict that you will make that choice), the feeling that accompanies the choosing is rarely perceived as being coerced. Therefore, when your mind is where you want it to be, you *feel* it is free, even though you may *believe* the choices that got you there were physically caused by preferences in your brain that you learned or inherited.

The bottom line of this thinking-feeling theory of free will is that the thinking that produces a belief in hard determinism seems to go with the feeling of freedom during the act of choosing, while the thinking that produces a belief in random choice seems to go with the feeling of coercion.

The foregoing remarks serve only to suggest how the resonating apical dendrite could relate to the problem of free will when making decisions. The issue of free will has a long history in scientific and philosophical inquiry, and free will deserves a more lengthy consideration than is allowed by the space given to it here.

Chapter 7

The Learning of Familiarity and Skills

"I don't know his name, but the face is familiar."

All of us have had that awkward moment when we instantly recognize a face, yet we can't come up with the name. Connecting names to people and places is the kind of memory stored by a network of connections, but instantly remembering a face or a place seems like a different kind of memory. Could a loop circuit store the face of a parent and a house lived in? This chapter shows that a loop circuit is as suitable for storing a visual impression of a face as a network circuit is suited for storing the connection of a name to a face.

The Process of Growing
Familiarity with an Apical Dendrite Cluster

So far in this book, the active apical dendrite has been pictured as a yellow cylinder. But many apical dendrites have a history of never being active. Tracing the growth of familiarity from its beginning typically requires a representation of the apical dendrite when it has never been activated. Figure 6.8 shows a cluster of apical dendrites in a loop circuit with active apical dendrites (colored yellow) surrounded by never-activated apical dendrites (with a light grey color). The grey apical dendrites look like tall empty jars in a fruit cannery waiting to be filled with yellow-colored lemonade. In this diagram, grey-colored apical dendrites change in color to yellow as they begin to receive pulses from the thalamus. Apical dendrites receive these pulses at the top, where the apical dendrite spreads its vine-like arbor very widely (see the tops of the apical dendrites shown in Figure 3.7). The arbors of adjacent apical dendrites intertwine, so that all apical dendrites located along a straight line of about 10 apical dendrites share contacts with each other. Thus, the view from above a cluster of apical dendrites will show a canopy of tiny interlaced fibers that resembles the view of a vine-covered sitting area outside a home. The lacework of these fibers actually extends everywhere along the surface of the human cortex because the tops of pyramidal neurons are spread out like overlapping umbrellas near the surface of the cerebral cortex.

Each point of contact between the tops of the many pyramidal neurons in this lacework of fibers can become a synapse. When the thalamus sends pulses to the top of a pyramidal neuron, it will facilitate the formation of a new synapse at a contact between two of these dendrites if the voltage at their point of contact is briefly increased to a high level[1]. The way that a rise in voltage usually happens is by shifting each pulse from one spike to a burst of several spikes (see Figure 6.1). The previous chapter pointed out that bursts of spikes occur during attention, and the intensity of a neural pulse made up of a burst of spikes can be increased by increasing the number of spikes in each burst.

Figure 7.1 illustrates the learning effect on a cluster of apical dendrites when something is perceived with a high level of attention. When inactive (colored grey) apical dendrites are recruited by the core of active apical dendrites (colored yellow), the number of active apical dendrites increases, as shown in Figure 7.2. The way an inactive apical

Attention Promotes Learning of
New Apical Dendrites

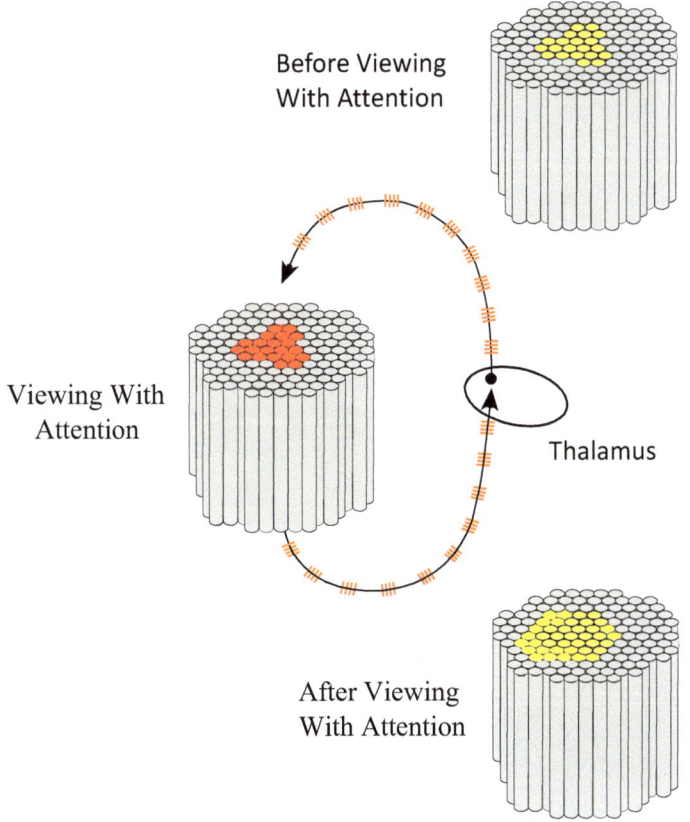

Before Viewing
With Attention

Viewing With
Attention

Thalamus

After Viewing
With Attention

Figure 7.1

The Growth of Familiarity

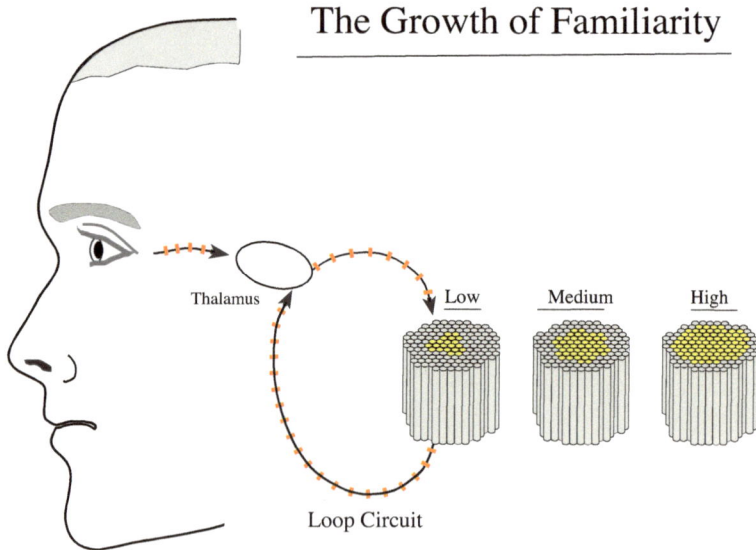

Figure 7.2

dendrite learns to be active is by the synaptic learning that underlies the way we learn the name of a flower. A condition for creating a synapse or for making an existing synapse stronger is to produce a brief rise of the intensity of rhythmic firing at the synapse[1]. In a recent 2018 experiment[2], a brief increase in the intensity of rhythmic firing at the synapse was also found to be one condition for learning within a short apical dendrite located in the touch region of the cortex. One way to promote this increase in firing is by the burst firing of attention.

This 2018 experiment[3] showed that the strengthening of a synapse on a short pyramidal apical dendrite in the touch area requires not only an increase in activity (voltage) in that neuron but also a blocking of inhibitory fibers that had previously prevented that apical dendrite from being activated. This disinhibition (inhibition of inhibition) component of strengthening a synapse on a short pyramidal neuron in a sensory area contrasts with the way that the strengthening of a synapse takes place in the network circuits of the hippocampus.

The blocking of inhibition in sensory learning is a different way of strengthening a synapse compared to the much-researched way that the hippocampus strengthens synapses in network circuits. The sensory area of touch is the area that shows evidence for the learning of many manual skills (to be described later in this chapter). We are assuming here that the brief elevation of intensity (voltage) at the synapse, which is necessary for learning of simple associations in the hippocampus and also for the learning of short pyramidal apical dendrites in the touch area of the cortex, extends to the learning of the long pyramidal apical dendrite in this area of the cortex. Further research is needed to confirm that this method of synaptic strengthening for short pyramidal apical dendrites also takes place for the long pyramidal apical dendrites of a sensory area, but this seems very likely because of the similar structure of these two kinds of pyramidal neurons.

To summarize the previous section, a high intensity of attention is assumed to promote the conversion of a never-active apical dendrite to an active apical dendrite, which strengthens the learning of familiarity of an object such as a face. The newly active apical dendrite can now be activated by the thalamus in the loop circuit. Even after these loops are established, the synaptic contacts with already active apical dendrites can be made stronger and more numerous when repetitions of the perception are also accompanied by attention.

An example of something seen with and without attention is the familiar painting that has been hanging in the hallway of your home for many years. You may notice its presence every time you walk by it (involving apical dendrites with a yellow code), but you do not stop to give it your attention. Hence, a daily glance at the painting does not increase its level of familiarity for you. But when you show the painting to a guest, you find yourself giving it the high level of attention that your guest is giving it, and this time your viewing of the painting will increase its familiarity for you.

Looking at the familiarity-learning topic with another example, neuroscientists believe that the recognition of faces is "special," because the process of recognizing faces is influenced by more factors than in recognizing other objects[4]. Nevertheless, it seems appropriate in the context of this book to ask whether or not familiarity for faces decays after a period of time. There is little evidence that clearly supports decay after age 70, but there is evidence that supports a decline in recognition accuracy after age 70. However, the kinds of errors made by the elderly in recognizing a face suggest that recognizing a face for them is vulnerable to interference from other faces in their memory; also, social influences at the time of recognition may play a role. So, according to current research, if a person fails to recognize a face that was once familiar, this does not necessarily indicate that some of the apical dendrites in the memory of the face have decayed or disappeared, but rather it suggests that other factors may have come into play. The number of loops representing similar things may increase to a point that they interfere with the act of remembering a particular face.

The growth of familiarity of a face, object, painting, melody, new taste or smell, or the feelings that a new friend gives you, all of these and more can be represented by increasing the size of the yellow core in a cluster (see Figure 7.2). Sometimes the cluster of activated apical dendrites produced by a perception can run out of never-activated (grey-colored) apical dendrites in its neighborhood because other perception-clusters have recruited them into their own clusters. When this crowding of clusters happens, the way that one cluster can continue to increase its size is by annexing apical dendrites from neighboring clusters, which reduces the number of apical dendrites in that neighboring cluster. This takeover of neighboring territories may be part of a decline in recognizing familiar faces. It may also be part of the reason that individuals with a highly learned mental skill sometimes show less than normal performance in other kinds of skills.

There is another way that a cluster of active apical dendrites can increase its number, and that is by the creation of new pyramidal neurons, each with its one apical dendrite. This availability of new neurons, called neurogenesis, appears to take place up to age 14 in the learning of music skills.

Growing Familiarity in Musical Skills

In 1995, a team of researchers investigated the responses of neurons in the cortex of musicians who played the violin, cello, or guitar[5]. The little finger in the left hand of string players is more involved in playing music than the thumb, and the little finger and thumb of the left hand are more active than the little finger and thumb of the right hand. Would the cortical area that represents the little finger of the left hand of musicians be larger than the area that represents the thumb? And would it be larger in the right hemisphere of the brain that represents the left hand than in the left hemisphere that represents the right hand? Finally, if these differences in cortical area are found for musicians, do all these differences disappear for non-musicians?

Understanding this experiment can be made easier by observing a map of the cortex that contains the regions that represent the fingers and the thumb. Figures 7.3 and 7.4 show cutaway views of the inside of the brain in the region where touch is felt at each point of the body surface. Note that the right side of Figure 7.3 represents the right hemisphere, and the left side represents the left hemisphere. In these figures the darker-grey ribbon on the outside of the brain shows the cortex (recall that in other images in this book, the cortex was colored blue), and the lighter-grey interior indicates the many long axons that connect distant parts of the cortex with each other. Figure 7.4 shows a map of the right side of the human body which is laid out along the top of the cortex that indicates where each small spot of the left side of the body sends pulses when it is touched. In this map, the sizes of the hand and fingers are shown larger than the other parts of the body surface because the number of neurons serving these areas is larger. Touching these areas with the tip of a pencil shows us that they are more sensitive than other areas to small changes in location of the pencil tip.

String players use the fingers of the left hand to produce the pitches of music, while the thumb is relatively inactive. Figure 7.5 shows the spots that represent the little finger and thumb in the right hemisphere. These two locations can be observed in Figure 7.4 at the two ends of the short horizontal strip of the cortex located below the drawing of the hand. The locations for the little finger and thumb of the right hand are in the same relative locations in the left hemisphere. Neural activity at these four locations in the cortex provided the results of the 1995 experiment. In this experiment, nine string players and six non-musicians received a small pressure on the little finger or thumb of each hand, which was delivered by a mechanical stimulator to ensure precise control and consistency in intensity and duration. The area of touch was small and located where the finger or thumb would touch a string on a violin, cello, or guitar (although the thumb does not usually touch a string during the normal playing of any of these instruments). A magnetic wave

The Touch Region for Parts of the Body Is Located Across the Top of a Cortical Slice Near the Center of the Brain

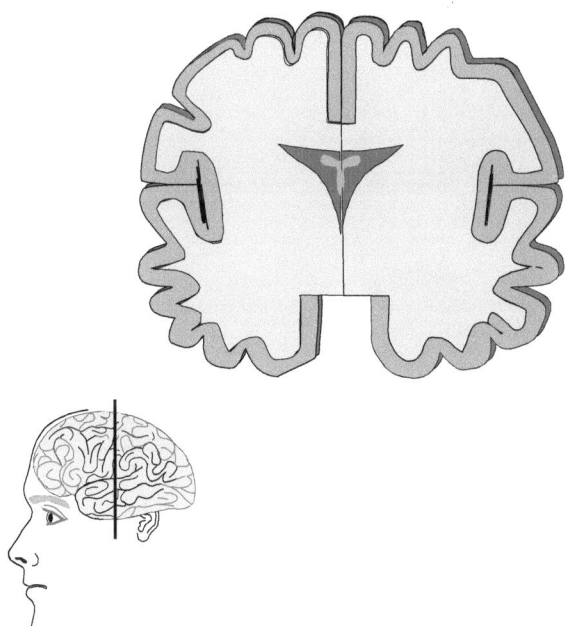

Figure 7.3

Map of the Surface of the Body
On a Slice of the Cortex

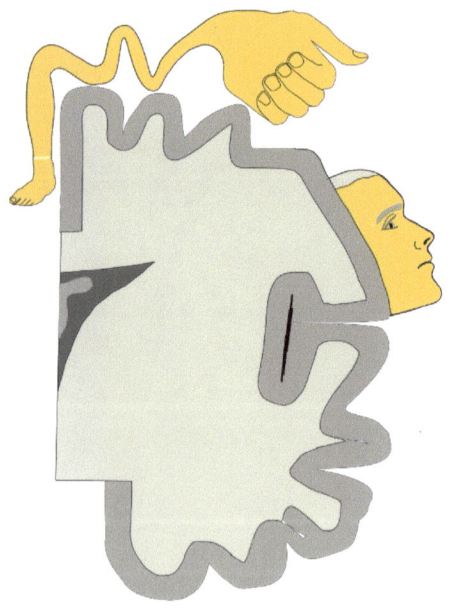

Figure 7.4

recorder was positioned over the head in the area where the cortical representations of the little finger and thumb are located.

A measurement device called the MEG (magneto-encephalogram) was used to record the number of electric dipoles at the little finger and thumb locations. An MEG measures the intensity of a magnetic field generated by a cluster of apical dendrites and can pinpoint with considerable accuracy the location of that activity. Recall from Chapter 5 that the apical dendrite dipole has opposite electric charges at both ends, and that a vibrating apical dendrite involves the shifting of electric charges between the top to the bottom of the apical dendrite (see Figure 5.1).

The longer the apical dendrite, the greater the intensity of its electric field, and since movements of an electric charge generates a magnetic field, an MEG record makes it possible to measure the magnitude of the electric dipole at each location in the brain. The magnitude of the measured electric dipole then can be used to estimate the number of pyramidal neurons (each with its apical dendrite) that contribute to the overall dipole of the cluster.

The estimated numbers of apical dendrites in the cortical areas serving the little finger and the thumb are represented by the areas of the circles shown in Figure 7.5. This figure shows electrical activity in the touch areas of little finger and thumb of musicians as black circles, and for those of the non-musicians as yellow circles. The magnitude of electrical activity in the area for the little finger is about twice as large for musicians compared to non-musicians. The authors of this study estimated that this difference in the electrical activity for the location of the little finger can be explained if about twice as many pyramidal neurons were active in musicians than were active in the non-musicians.

Earlier in this chapter it was mentioned that when new apical dendrites are created, they expand the hills and a deepen the valleys in the part of the cortical surface in which the neurogenesis takes place. This distortion of the surface of the cortex can often be observed without the aid of magnification. So, when a surgeon first sees the surface of the patient's brain in an open-brain operation the surgeon can quickly conclude whether or not the patient is a string player.

The brain of Albert Einstein was preserved for research, and it shows a visible "knob" of expansion in the surface of the same cortical area where string players show an expansion. Einstein studied the violin from age 6 to 14, and thereafter, according to his own report, he spent more time playing the violin than thinking about physics. Also, a large part of the back area of his brain (the parietal cortex), where spatial imaging is believed to take place, reveals a surface area that is not only larger than normal, but also has surface variations that give that area an overall unique appearance[6].

Growing Familiarity in Athletic Skills
Another study of skill learning that involves small areas of the cortex compared the hand and foot areas of handball players and ballet dancers[7]. Twelve professional ballet dancers and 10 professional handball players, all right-handed women whose average age was 24 years, received magnetic resonance brain scans (MRIs). The regions of interest are the hand and foot areas of the cortex, shown on the body surface-to-cortex map of Figure 7.6.

The results in Figure 7.6 show areas of the hand and foot for ballet dancers and for handball players. In this diagram, the sizes of the two black circles indicate that the foot areas of ballet dancers are larger than their hand areas, and the sizes of the two white circles indicate that the hand areas of handball players are larger than their foot areas. A comparison of the cortical areas for each skill shows that the foot areas are larger for ballet dancers and the hand areas are larger for handball players.

The two areas that are shown here reside in the sensory (touch) part of the cortex, but similar results were found for the motor (response) part of the cortex, which lies above the line (representing the large valley over the top of the cortex) and above the sensory parts. These findings show that ballet dancers have more cortical area devoted

Representations in the Brain of the Little Finger and Thumb:
Attentive Use Increases Their Cortical Areas

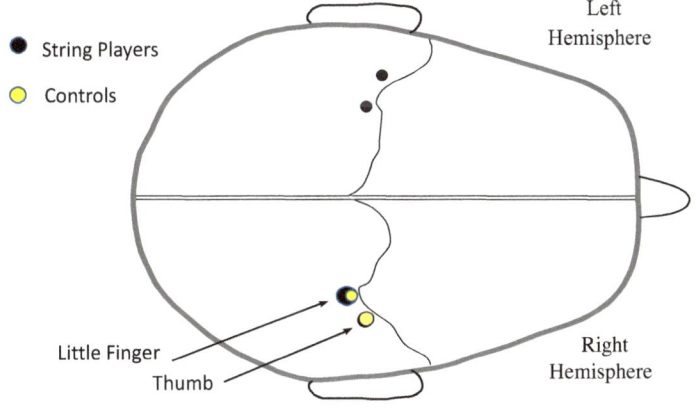

Figure 7.5

Representations in the Brain of the Foot And Hand: Attentive Use Increases Their Cortical Areas

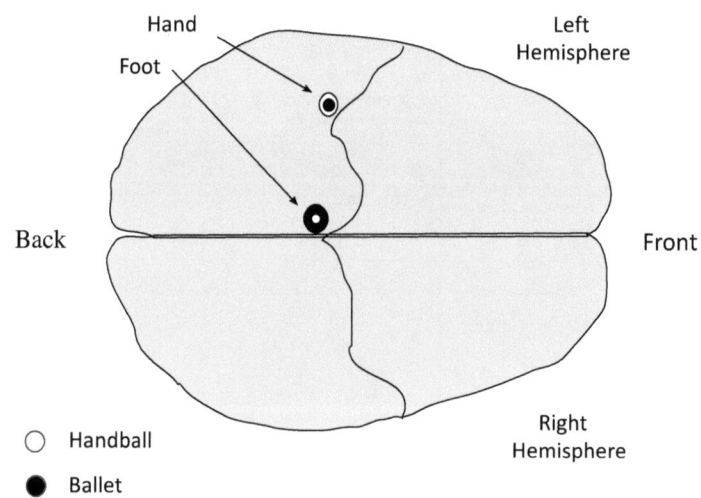

Figure 7.6

to foot movements and handball players have more area devoted to hand movements. It should be noted that since the participants in this study were all right-handed, the observed differences in cortical areas showed up only in their left hemispheres.

The interpretation of the results of the two studies just described is sometimes questioned because it is possible that the differences in cortical areas may have been produced by biological differences that existed before the measurements were made. Compared to the average person, a person born with talented finger dexterity may be more likely to choose to play a string instrument, and a person born with the body of a ballet dancer may be more likely to choose to study ballet.

Historical accounts of the childhood of highly talented individuals suggests a genetic gift of generous amounts of active apical dendrites in auditory and visual areas of the cortex. At the age of three, when he could barely reach the piano keyboard, Mozart would press a key that sounded one note, and only after listening to that note for a lengthy duration did he move his finger to sound another note. Frank Lloyd Wright wrote in his autobiography that at the age of six he spread colored pencils from a newly opened box across his hand to simply stare at them. When Dante was nine years old, he first gazed upon the face of the young Beatrice, with only passing glimpses of that face in the following few years before her early death. The first image of Beatrice was strong enough to inspire his highly visual writing of the *Divine Comedy*, a long poem begun at about the age 45 and completed a year before his death at the age of 56.

In an attempt to control for possible pre-existing differences between groups in the two experiments just described, a 2009 study[8] in Boston assigned six year olds who had no prior formal musical training to two groups which were matched by gender, age, and the socio-economic status of their parents. The "instrument" group received 15 months of weekly half-hour music lessons, and the "control" group received no instrumental music training during the 15-month period, but participated in a weekly 40-minute group music class that engaged in singing and playing with drums and bells. Each child received two magnetic resonance brain scans (MRIs): one at the beginning and one at the end of the 15-month activities. The MRI images from the two before-and-after brain scans showed spots of activity in the brain, and when the first activity image was subtracted from the second activity image the change in the intensity of a spot of activity could be measured. The images in Figures 7.7 and 7.8 show the locations of active spots in the brain along with the differences in intensity coded by color of the first and second scans. The lighter colored spots show higher levels of statistical significance, but all colored spots indicate an increase in size of areas of activity.

In the image of Figure 7.7 the spot of interest is located in the right precentral hill of the motor area. This area serves the action of moving the fingers. The finding that this area showed expansion suggests that the number of active pyramidal neurons and their apical dendrites within it increases in number as the actions of piano playing become more familiar. Since the children were randomly assigned to each training condition, the contribution of a genetic head-start in musical abilities can be ruled out.

In Figure 7.8, the spot of interest is located in Heschl's gyrus, which is a long hill buried within the brain slightly above the level of the ear. Neurons in this hill are the first in the cortex to receive electric pulses from the ear. The incoming pathways from the ear enter the thalamus and then are relayed to the network and loop circuits as shown (faintly) in Figure 7.8. The increase in the activity in this primary auditory area of the cortex implies that additional active pyramidal neurons and their apical dendrites have expanded the initial boundaries of this area. This finding indicates that the area of reception of incoming pulses from the thalamus has increased the brain's capacity to receive the sounds of music. So, it could be said that as we hear more music, we strengthen our ability to hear music and therefore we hear music more fully.

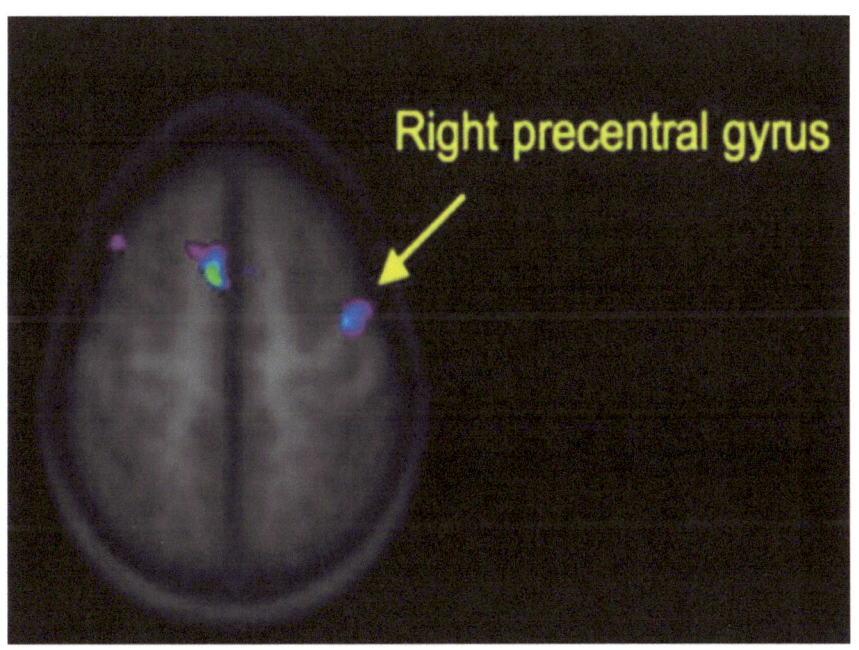

Figure 7.7

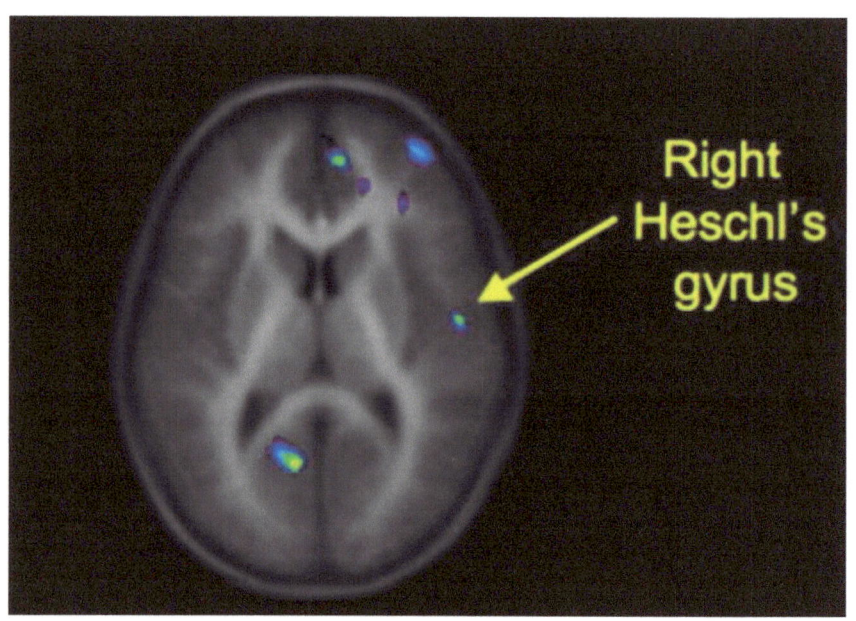

Figure
7.8

The central idea of this chapter is that the performance of athletic and musical skills involves active pyramidal apical dendrites in specific regions of the cortex that represent these skills. The evidence supporting the learning of skills is the increase in size of spots in particular sensory and motor areas of the cortex that are involved while performing the skill, which sometimes produces an expansion of cortical hills and a deepening of cortical valleys.

The learning of familiarity in the acquisition of skills and in the perception of music is assumed to be represented in the brain by the increase in the size of cortical spots in which clusters of apical dendrites are specialized for skills and perception of objects. Many of these memory clusters also support our abilities to *imagine* performing a skill or perceiving an object, according to the research of Kosslyn and his colleagues[9].

Memory Clusters of Apical Dendrites
that Represent What We Are Perceiving

For us perceptions are what **is**, but much of our mental life is spent in imagining what **could be**, from expectations of what is about to happen next in our daily routines to imagining how to create better social environments or how to create a new work of art. Our creating of these things usually begins with the cluster-based image of a familiar object or scene, and then we construct a modified version of that image. At first, the new image consists of a few apical dendrites, but the number of apical dendrites increases as we revisit the image and fill in more details.

Our imaging does not consist only of visualizations, which we produce when we read a story or when someone reads a story to us. We also produce images of sounds, especially when we hear tunes playing in our heads. We can imagine what objects feel like, what food tastes like, and sometimes we can imagine the smell of a rose.

The English poet and critic T.S. Eliot used a system of images in his poems to communicate a particular feeling to the reader. He called this system the *objective correlative* because it enabled him to use a word or small group of words to call up a specifie feeling. For example, the *yew tree* was intended to evoke the feeling of death, and the *rose garden* the feeling of Eden-like paradise. Wood of the yew tree was suitable for making bows, but the berries, needles, seeds, and bark are poisonous. In English history yew trees were usually found among graves in English churchyards where children and farm animals were unlikely to stray. Hence words that evoked an image of a yew also evoked the feeling of death.

Eliot said:

> *The only way of expressing emotion in the form of art is by finding an 'objective correlative'; in other words, a set of objects, a situation, a chain of events which shall be the formula of that particular emotion; such that when the external facts, which must terminate in sensory experience, are given, the emotion is immediately evoked* [11,12].

The link between an objective scene and the subjective feeling that it calls up is embodied in the loop connections between the clusters of apical dendrites that are active when we perceive or imagine an object (or scene) and the clusters that are active when we experience particular emotional feelings. Both the image and the emotional feeling are *experienceable* because they are based on vibrating loop circuits. In contrast, words that are heard or read are understood by the processing of network circuits. It is the poet's task to strengthen the links between the image of a scene and the emotion it evokes, usually by the literary method of "show, don't tell," which involves evoking images and feelings instead of "telling" (describing) the relations between the scene and an emotional response. By "showing" the images and feelings, the corresponding neural activities are both sustained for a time in the experiencing mode and consequently the opportunities for being associated are increased.

In the 18th and 19th century, the word *sensibility* was more likely to appear in books and journals than it is today. Regarded as a part of a person's character, sensibility was defined as the capacity for sensing and feeling and the ability to appreciate and respond to complex emotional or aesthetic influences. The most recent decline in the use of the word "sensibility" is apparently related to the decline in the use of the words *sensing* and *feeling*. Could one reason for this decline be that the rise of the information-processing view of mental activity tends to filter out concepts and ideas of mental activity that are not easily represented in the processing of computers? This chapter shows that the concept of sensing actions and musical patterns can be easily represented by clusters of apical dendrites in brain circuits, and the next chapter shows that feelings also can be easily represented by clusters of apical dendrites. Will this development in our knowledge of how the brain works lead to a re-emergence in our language of words like sensibility, which denote the capacity of individuals to sense their physical environments and to sense their feelings and the feeling of others?

Chapter 8

How Does the Brain
Produce an Intense Experience?

There are moments that seem so intense we think our life will never again be the same. Leaving our first family home, seeing your newborn child smile at you, standing in a place that is sacred to you, learning of the accidental death of your best friend, and graduating from school are all examples of special experiences that may change our outlook on life. Events like these can seize our attention and push it to a very high level of intensity and hold our attention for long durations of time in which we cannot think of anything else.

What is happening in the brain while we are experiencing such intense levels of attention? In particular, what are the loop circuits with their apical dendrites doing to elevate attention to such high levels? The study of intense attention in the laboratory is limited by the kinds of situations that can be brought to the laboratory setting, but there are other, more acceptable ways to raise the level of emotional feelings than the exceptional situations just described.

A particularly productive way to study emotional feelings in the laboratory is to observe the brain activity of individuals while they look at paintings. Brain scans are already available from many experiments of this kind. In a typical study, observers are asked to do a specific thing while they observe a painting, such as making a subjective judgment of their emotional feelings or making objective judgments about the objects in a painting. In order to discover what brain areas are most active, the brain scans from these experiments can be superimposed upon each other. First, the image of each individual brain is fit to a standard brain image, then combining the individual scans will reveal what areas are common to all of the scans while cancelling out areas that are active only in the scan contributed by one or two individuals.

A 2014 study[1] combined the MRI brain scans of individuals in 15 different experiments published between 2004 and 2012, all involving the viewing of paintings. In Figure 8.1 the composite brain scan is shown as a horizontal slice across the center of the brain. The active brain areas common to the participants in all 15 experiments included a very large visual area at the bottom of the brain slice of Figure 8.1 plus a cortical area that is active while having feelings (upper left), and a small area below the cortex (upper right) that is involved in storing the memory of a visual shape. The two areas that contain pyramidal neurons (with their apical dendrites) in loop circuits are the large visual area at the bottom of Figure 8.1 and the small feelings area in the upper left of that figure.

However, there is one important area of viewing a painting that does not show up in this composite scan, which is the area that controls attention. It is obvious that each task in the different experiments required attention, even though each task required attention to be directed to different things for each individual. In each of these 15 experiments the observers are instructed to respond to a painting in a particular way. For example, a viewer in the study may be shown a series of abstract and representational paintings and then asked to press one button when they recognize an object and press another button when no object is recognized. Or the viewer may be an expert who judges the

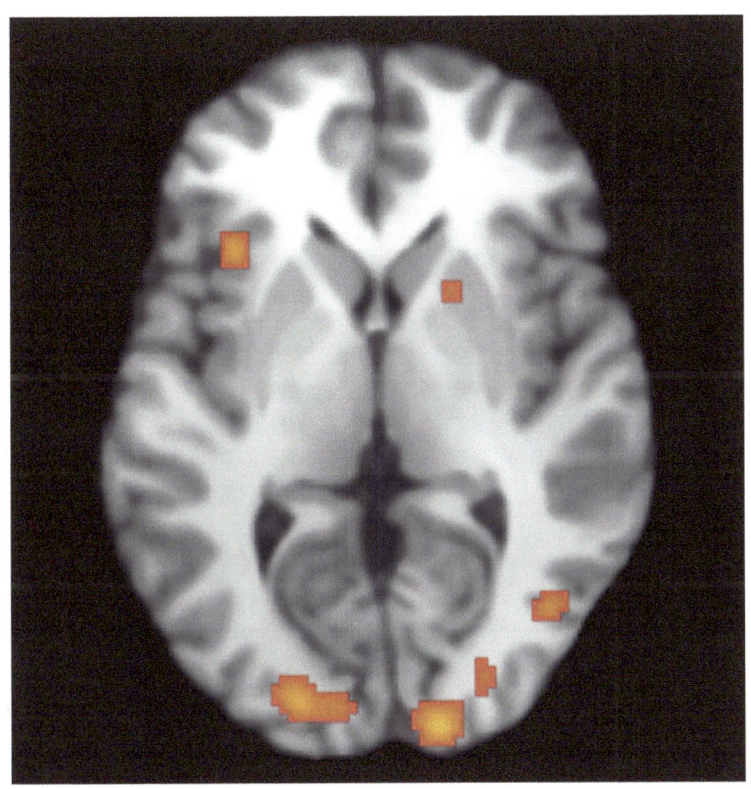

Figure 8.1

value of a painting when monetary favors are involved versus when no monetary favors are involved.

Each of the instructions described in the preceding paragraph prompted a viewer to attend to the paintings in a specific way that may have engaged different specific parts of the relatively large attention area. So, when the scans of the different experiments were superimposed into a composite scan, no single part of the attention area would be active enough to show up on the composite brain scan. In order to obtain a single, more sensitive measure of attention activity only one experiment was chosen for further analysis.

One experiment in the group of 15 experiments, the 2009 experiment[2], instructed the viewers to direct their attention to the paintings in one of two ways: either "to approach the images in an objective and detached manner to obtain information about the content of the painting," or "to approach the paintings in a subjective and engaged manner, experiencing the mood of the work and the feelings it evokes, and to focus on its colors, tones, composition, and shapes." The first instruction was called the "pragmatic" condition and the second instruction was called the "aesthetic" condition. Thus there were two brain scans for each painting, and by superimposing one scan over the other scan, the resulting scan showed the areas of the brain that changed their activity levels when the one instruction changed to the other instruction.

The brain scans in Figure 8.2 show areas where there were statistically significant differences between the aesthetic and pragmatic scans (note that in Figure 8.2, the letters R and L are displayed in mirror image, in order to correct for a convention to reverse the right and left sides in presenting scan images).

The scan image in Figure 8.2B shows activations in the visual areas (at the bottom) and in the areas of emotional feeling (at the upper left), which are consistent with the results of the 2014 study (described above) that showed composite scans from the 15 different experiments. The authors also tested whether the experience of emotion plays a

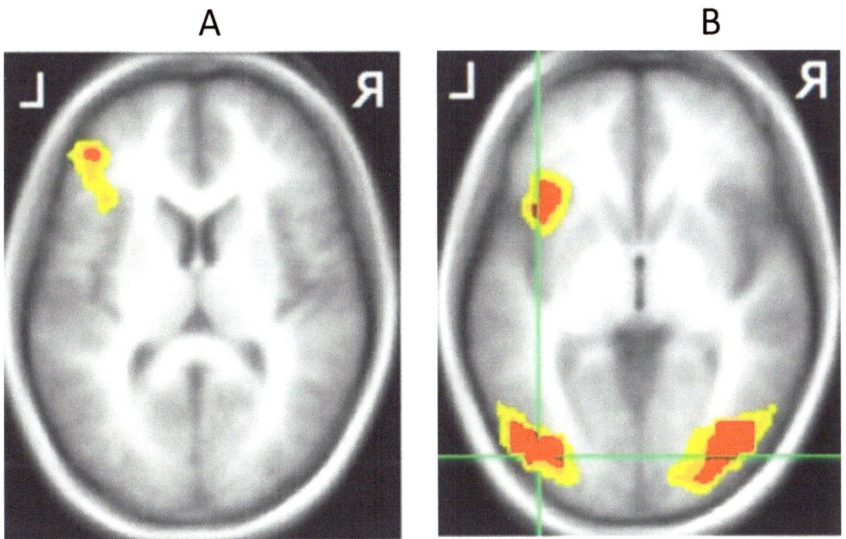

Figure 8.2

larger role in the aesthetic condition than in the pragmatic condition. A comparison of the brain scans gave a positive answer to this question for the emotional feeling areas on both sides of the brain.

Subtracting the pragmatic scan from the aesthetic scan revealed a small area at the upper left corner of Figure 8.2A, which confirmed the hypothesis that the area of attention control in viewing paintings of this experiment is located in the left prefrontal cortex, an area in the front part of the brain well-known to serve the control of visual attention to visual objects.

Taken together, the results of the brain scans of the 2009 experiment, shown on both sides of Figure 8.2, support the hypothesis that three particular areas of the cortex show increased activity whenever a painting is viewed with some purpose in mind, ranging from the pragmatic purpose of obtaining information to the aesthetic purpose of experiencing subjective feelings. These areas are the visual area, the feelings area, and the area of attention control shown by the drawing in Figure 8.3.

The results suggest that the visual area, attention control area, and the feelings area work together to produce the wide differences in reactions to a particular painting from one person to another. Individuals differ in the size of a particular area of active apical dendrites after special training (see Figures 7.5, 7.6, 7.7, 7.8), and it seems reasonable to expect individuals to differ over their life spans in virtually all cortical areas serving mental activity. Finding two individuals, even identical twins, who show exactly the same sizes of active apical dendrite areas for visual processing, feelings, and attention-control seems highly unlikely.

The many ways in which these three areas can influence each other can be examined with the aid of the diagrams in Figure 8.3 and Figure 8.4. Figure 8.4 provides details of the connections between loop circuits from the three major cortical areas and shows a theoretical diagram of the locations of three main areas that the 2009 and 2014 studies found to be active while individuals observed paintings (see Figures 8.1 and

8.2). The loop circuit on the lower right part of Figures 8.3 and 8.4 corresponds to the loop circuit in Figure 3.4, where pulses from the eye contact a neuron in the thalamus, which is part of the circuit loop that activates an apical dendrite in the visual sensation area of the cortex.

The visual area in the human brain is very large, and it includes many smaller areas that participate in the early cortical stages of processing a visual object. Therefore, Figures 8.3 and 8.4 have been simplified to show only one cluster for visual sensation. Thus, using the drawings in Figure 8.3 and 8,4 one can easily locate the locations of clusters of apical dendrites in the visual area, the feelings area, and the attention area along with the three loops that connect the three areas. Figure 8.4 shows the locations of connections between the three loops (where the tips of the arrows intersect a loop inside the thalamus). Each cluster of apical dendrites represents hundreds of thousands of apical dendrites.

Figure 8.4 indicates that a connection between two clusters of apical dendrites is not a direct one, but instead is formed by connecting their loop circuits to a neuron within the thalamus (the neuron is located where the point of an arrow contacts a loop).

Note that in Figure 8.3, the neurons within the thalamus are not shown for clarity so that the main point of the figure can be distinctly shown, which is that two loops connect with each other via the thalamus and not directly by a direct loop-to-loop synapse. In network circuits, neurons commonly connect directly with each other. But neurons in separate loop circuits do not connect directly with each other. Instead, their loop circuits connect indirectly with each other at synapses in the thalamus (as shown in Figure 8.4). Therefore, it appears that there are two major ways to functionally connect neurons in separate brain areas to each other, one for network circuits and another for loop circuits.

These two ways of connecting neurons, indirectly through their chain of loops or directly between their network circuits, implies that the learning of these connections may take place in different ways.

Unconnected Loop Circuits With Bundles of Apical Dendrites

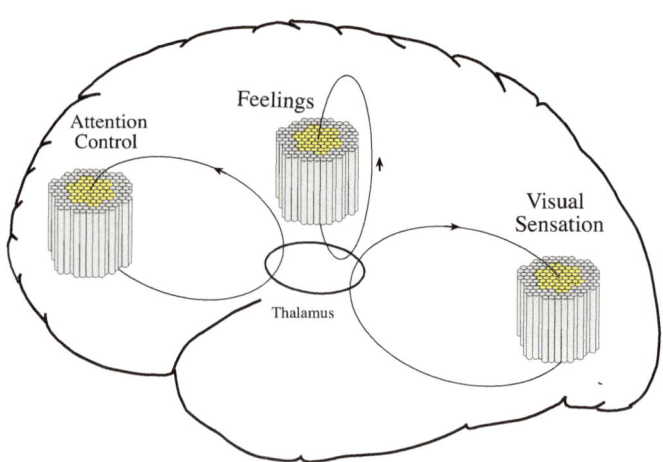

Figure 8.3

Connected Loop Circuits With Bundles of
Apical Dendrites

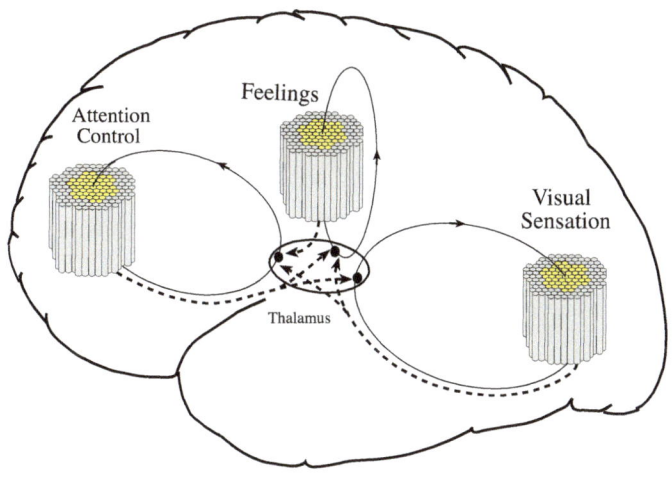

Figure 8.4

Consequently, a disease that weakens one kind of synaptic learning (e.g., in a network connection) may not affect the other kind of synaptic learning (e.g., in a loops connection). For example, the neural disorders that produce the forgetting of recent conversations in Alzheimer's disease may not affect the memory of a recently learned skill[3].

The cluster of apical dendrites in the feelings area can be activated to several different levels of intensity by the cluster in the attention area. These levels are indicated by the colors yellow, orange, and red in Figures 6.2 and 6.9. The change in activity level of the feelings cluster is also strongly influenced by the reward value of viewing the painting, whose source is in a subcortical area[4,5].

The usual cycle of stimulating the three areas in the brain begins with looking at a painting (see Figures 8.3 and 8.4). The visual sensation cluster is activated first, and then it activates the feeling and attention clusters by activating their loops via synapses in the thalamus. The visual sensation cluster also sends fibers into the regions below the cortex that represent the reward value of looking at the painting (as noted above). Fibers from these subcortical regions then return activation to the feeling loop that affects the activity level of the feelings cluster in the cortex.

The feelings cluster, in turn, sends fibers that increase the activity level of the loop of the attention cluster, which then increases the activity level in the loop of the visual sensation cluster. The sensation cluster then sustains the activation levels in the feelings and attention circuits by returning activation to these two levels. The sensation cluster can raise the level of its own returning activations, which amounts to positive feedback by its loop circuit. Large sizes of the feelings and attention clusters can do the same. In this way, feedback loops can produce a very high level of activation of all three clusters which results in a very intense level of experiencing of an object, an experience which seems to "fill the mind."

Several examples of intense experiences that seem to "fill the mind" were given at the beginning of this chapter. One way to understand the participation of apical dendrites in producing these kinds of experiences is by referring to the diagrams of Figures 8.3 and 8.4.

Figures 8.3 and 8.4 show clusters of apical dendrites that produce three major aspects of a visual experience: the ongoing visual impressions, the feelings produced, and the strength and intensity of attention to these impressions and feelings. The understanding of this experiencing builds on the information from previous chapters. For example, Figure 6.2 shows the various levels of attention that can influence experiencing the appearance of objects such as paintings. Figure 7.1 shows how the strength of each of these three clusters can be increased through learning. According to the present theory, the probability of adding new active apical dendrites to a cluster will be increased when the intensity of attention is raised, and the larger the cluster of apical dendrites the higher the potential level of intensity of that cluster.

An example from the *Divine Comedy*, a 14th century poem by Dante, may help illuminate the ways that the three clusters in Figures 8.3 and 8.4 combine their activities to elevate an experience to a very high level. In the last verse of the the *Divine Comedy*, Dante described the greatest experience of gazing at a light that he could imagine with these words, translated here from Italian to English[6]:

> *So, with my mind completely suspended*
> *and my gaze fixed, unmoving, and attentive,*
> *the gazing kept increasing the intensity*
> *of the act of gazing.*
> *That light was such that to turn from it to any*
> *other sight was impossible for me to consent to.*

Apparently, in this description of an intense experience, the act of attending to the light is being intensified even while the observer is gazing at the light. This increase in the level of attention, according to the diagram in Figure 8.4, is produced when the resonating activity in the visual cluster is being passed along to the feelings cluster, and then to the attention cluster via connections between the loops that contain the clusters. The connection between the cluster of attention and the cluster of visual resonating serves to maintain the current level of activities in the attention and visual clusters. In order to increase that level, however, the attention cluster must receive additional activation, which is provided by the input from the feelings cluster. Repeating such an experience will add new apical dendrites to the visual and attention clusters, so that the intensity of looking at that light can increase to even higher levels.

In this manner, each of the three loops acts as a positive feedback loop, and each of the clusters contributes to the strength of its loop when the number of its active apical dendrites is increased by repeated occasions of use. The learning process that produces the increase in apical dendrites is assumed to be promoted at those moments when the level of attention in the loop circuits is high, and the level of attention in all three loops moves upward as long as the positive feedback activity continues.

How high an intensity of a particular experience can be reached depends, of course, on the size of the bursts produced by the attention loop, but it also depends on inputs from motivation and reward areas located below the cortex, whose levels may be influenced by genetic factors. Also, how high the intensity can go depends on the sizes of the three relevant clusters, which, in turn depend on the number of available apical dendrites in the cortical neighborhoods that can be recruited into each cluster by learning. There seems to be no research to provide an estimate of the upper limit of pyramidal neurons (with their apical dendrites) that could be recruited to increase the size of a cluster shown in Figures 8.3 and 8.4.

Previous discussion in Chapter 7 described the annexing of neighboring apical dendrites that serve other mental content. It is conceivable that dedicated experiencing of one object (e.g., playing a guitar) could eventually take over or annex most of the apical dendrites in the cortical vicinity of the initial memory clusters, which potentially could weaken the original level of functioning served by the cortical areas that lose apical dendrites to the annexation. Another source of new apical dendrites lies in neurogenesis, which adds more areas to the existing surface of a cortical area and extends the peaks and deepens the valleys of the cortex.

Further comments about the limits of intense experiences would be reaching even further from what can currently be supported by experimental data. But it is hard to ignore the apparent existence of large amounts of untapped cortical tissue in the areas serving vision, feeling, and attention. These supplies of yet-to-be-activated apical dendrites suggest that many individuals can continue to increase the heights and fullness of experiences that their brains can give them. Figure 8.5 illustrates how repeated experiencing of a painting[7] can prepare an observer for a fuller and more intense experience of that painting.

In summary, this chapter focuses on the activities of three areas of the cortex during the experience of gazing at an object. The learning of active apical dendrites was illustrated by the increase in the size of a cluster, so that the gradual preparation for a fuller experience of a particular object of art is produced by the progressive increase of active apical dendrites in the feeling cluster and in the attention control clusters as well as in the cluster size of visual sensations of that object. This increase in the level of neural learning depends not only on the existing number of apical dendrites (active and inactive), but also on the less understood number of pyramidal neurons that may be created anew by neurogenesis. Growing more pyramidal neurons with their active apical dendrites not only makes it possible to experience a painting more fully, but also to more fully experience a melody of music, a line of poetry, the face of a friend, and the vast array of stars in the night sky.

Preparing the Mind/Brain for Viewing a Work of Art

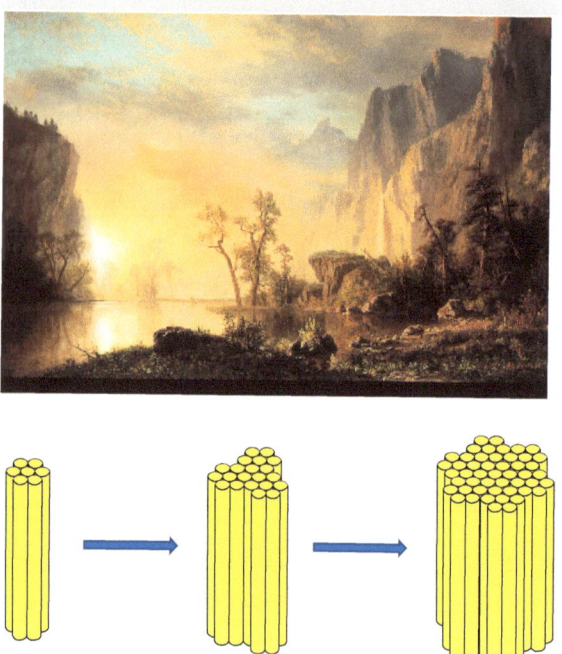

Figure 8.5

Chapter 9

The Role of the Insula
in the Experiencing of Feelings

The word *feelings* as used in this book describes the particular kind of experiences common to pleasure, pain, love, cravings, addictions, musical enjoyment, eating, and general well-being. Hence, feelings not only refer to the intense experiences of emotion but also to the many experiences that are less intense than the states we call *emotion*.

A part of the cortex that is active during the experiencing of emotional feelings, and the feelings that were discussed in the previous paragraph is the *insula*, shown in Figure 9.1 as a thumb-sized structure that lies out of sight when viewing the brain, and is located above and slightly in front of the ear in both hemispheres of the brain. For the purposes of this book, the insula may be divided into three parts: front, middle, and back (anterior, intermediate, and posterior insula).

The kinds of neurons found in each of these three parts of the insula are especially important because long pyramidal neurons in layers 5 and 6 of the insula cortex indicate the presence of loop circuits, and stellate neurons in layer 4 indicate inputs to network circuits. In the insula, the back part contains both kinds of neurons, and the front part appears to

The Insula

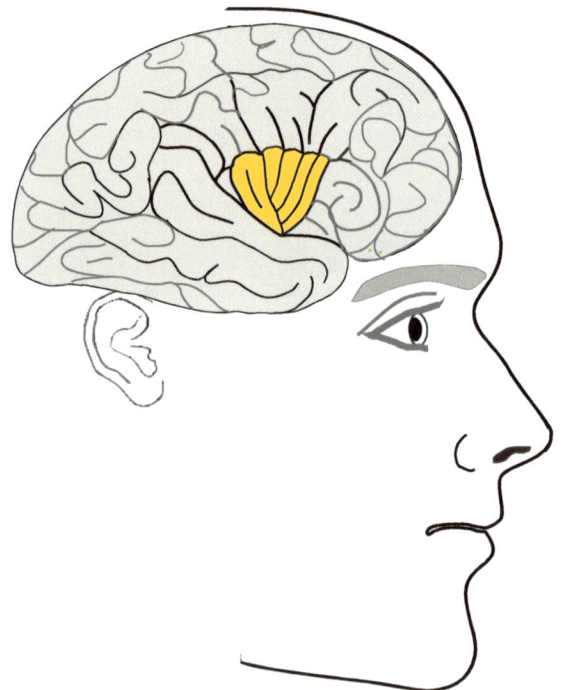

The Insula Revealed by Pulling Back Frontal and Temporal Cortices

Figure 9.1

contain only long neurons, while the middle part contains pyramidal neurons plus a smaller and smaller number of stellate neurons as it approaches its border with the front part[1]. Therefore, moving from the back part to the front part of the insula produces mental activities that contain less and less informational content.

The apparent absence of stellate neurons and horizontal connections in the front part of the insula suggests that the front part of the insula (henceforth labeled the frontal insula) is not devoted to processing information about particular feelings but rather devoted to experiencing feelings. The circuitry in the back part of the insula resembles the circuitry in a region of the adjacent somatosensory (touch) area, which maps the parts of the body (see Figure 7.4). When an object touches the side of the face, the experience of the sensation is accompanied by information about the location, pressure, temperature, and sometimes even the general outline of the object. So, the mental effect of activating the back part of the insula contains network-based information that makes it easy to detail what you just felt. In contrast, a sudden increase in the speed of a descending elevator can produce a sensation that is accompanied by relatively little information. As a result, the frontal insula is activated, and because it contains little or no network of stellate neurons, the feeling you just had resists description and makes it difficult to describe what you just felt.

One might suggest that the French impressionist paintings of the 19th century stimulated the brains of viewers in a manner that moved the activation of the insula away from the traditional perception of the details in paintings that are represented at the back end of the insula toward experiencing paintings more as formless impressions, represented at the front end of the insula. Meditation experiments[6] show that when expert meditators are attending to their feelings of compassion for others, it is their frontal insula that is more active than the frontal insula of novice meditators.

In view of these considerations, one could say that the mental effect of an activated frontal insula is a subjective impression. Clues concerning what other cortical areas produce this kind of activation can be gathered from knowing what areas send their fibers to the frontal insula, and from inspecting the external objects or events that prompted this activity in the brain.

As described earlier, apical dendrites of pyramidal neurons are activated by a series of pulses carried by the axons that contact the apical dendrite at its top location (see Figure 3.4). These pulses produce the electric vibration in the apical dendrite, which causes the cell body to discharge a steady series of spikes in the output axon of the neuron. In the case of the frontal insula, this output apparently is almost always sent to a thalamic neuron, and from there returns to the top of the apical dendrite in a loop circuit.

The axons that provide trains of steady pulses to pyramidal neurons (and their apical dendrites) in the frontal insula apparently arise from neurons in the thalamus, and not from neurons in networks. These thalamic neurons, in turn, receive their steady inputs from several other areas. Among these areas are those that are activated by internal organs of the body that produce "gut feelings" from whatever we are currently sensing.

Another source of steady pulses is the subcortical amygdala, which "orchestrates" how the internal organs of the body react during intense emotions, especially fear. While on a hike, the sight of a large snake in your path very quickly produces "emergency" reactions of the heart, lungs, stomach, and adrenal glands. This fast track to survival owes its speed to the fact that it is routed through the reflexes of the amygdala instead of through the deliberative, attention-controlled circuits of the cortex. The amygdala also sends a steady train of pulses directly to the frontal insula, which produces the feelings that accompany the sight of the snake. In an attempt to capture this feeling, we often report "what it is like" to be walking along a path and suddenly see a large snake.

The feeling of fright, in this example, is normally not localized in one part of the body, but instead seems to involve the whole body. Another whole-body feeling is the uneasiness experienced while walking in a crowd. Milder examples are how you feel when you relax in a comfortable chair after a meal or right after you have solved a difficult problem. Perhaps the most familiar example of a whole-body feeling comes to you when someone simply asks, "How are you feeling?" [2]

The frontal insula, then, is involved with experiencing intense feelings of emotions as well as milder feelings that accompany pleasurable and uncomfortable events of daily life. In most moments of daily life feelings have a low intensity, and they are labeled simply as feelings. Examples of low-intensity feelings usually arise in us when we listen to music or visit a museum. These are the most convenient kinds of feelings to measure in laboratory experiments.

An experimental study in 2011 [3] found that an area located above the eyes (the orbitofrontal cortex, an area known to control attention to feelings) was more active when individuals listened to a piece of music or viewed a picture that they previously had rated as beautiful. Their brain activity was compared to that of individuals who were indifferent to these works of art. The results also showed that the strength of the activation in this cortical area increased as the rating of beauty increased.

In a 2008 experiment involving meditation [4], investigators measured activity of the insula using fMRI while novice and expert practitioners of meditation generated a loving-kindness-compassion meditation state. During meditation, activation in the insula was greater during presentation of negative sounds (of distress) than positive or neutral sounds in expert meditators than it was in novice meditators.

Variations in the Volume of the Frontal Insula of Individuals

As noted before, the frontal insula is made up mostly of pyramidal neurons and a small number of inhibitory neurons. Therefore, changes in the total cortical volume of this area would appear to indicate changes in the number of pyramidal neurons within it, along with their apical dendrites.

The number of pyramidal neurons in a cortical area can be estimated by measuring the volume of the cortex. A 2004 article [5] used MRI to estimate the volume of the frontal insula while people were judging the timing of their own heartbeats. The authors observed that the volume of cortical gray matter in the frontal insula increased as their timing accuracy increased. The volume also increased as their subjective rating of awareness of their internal organs increased.

The increase in numbers of pyramidal neurons in a cortical area was addressed earlier in Chapter 7 of this book with respect to the expansion of cortical areas of touch and movement involved in learning to play a string instrument, such as a violin or guitar. According to the Loops Theory, a gain in surface area is caused by adding more pyramidal neurons (with their long apical dendrites) to the already active pyramidal neurons. The way a new pyramidal neuron joins an existing cluster of these neurons is by activating these neurons to a level of intensity that is high enough to produce burst firing. High levels of activation are produced by high levels of attention.

Attending to Feelings

As mentioned above, the directing of attention to the frontal insula is believed to activate the cortical area located above the eye (the same place that increases its activity level when individuals rate the beauty of music and paintings). Apparently, this area also controls our attention to sensations of feelings that arise from responses of the internal organs. According to a 1984 study[6], the activation of this orbitofrontal area of attention control causes its pyramidal neurons to send burst pulses to the thalamic neuron in a loop circuit, and that thalamic neuron, in turn, sends burst pulses in another loop circuit to pyramidal neurons in the frontal insula. These two loop circuits form a chain whose two links (loops) are joined by a common thalamic neuron. By means of this chain of loop circuits, the attention control area above the eye boosts the electric vibrations in the frontal insula to raise the intensity of the feeling.

This is where the *hub circuit structure* enters the story. The hub spreads the activation of the frontal insula to many cortical and subcortical areas.

The insula has been described as a hub of connections to the many cortical areas that support the mental activities in the brain[7]. A hub works by bringing together in one place connections from several cortical areas. When one input to the hub is active, the output of the hub to other areas become activated so that the activation in the initiating area is spread widely to other areas. Hence, the hub operations for loop circuits are particularly effective in expanding electric vibrations from one cortical area to several other cortical areas.

The hub of the frontal insula is special because it apparently contains only pyramidal neurons. The long pyramidal neurons located here vibrate electrically while network activity appears to be absent. This finding was reported in a 2019 article[8] that also provides a detailed description of the anatomy of the insula, along with a model of how it functions.

To summarize this section, when the frontal insula is activated from the cortical area above the eye, its pyramidal neurons send streams of steady pulses to many thalamic neurons via loop circuits, and these thalamic neurons, in turn, send streams of pulses in loop circuits to many widely separated cortical and subcortical areas. Some of these areas serve cognitive functions, while others serve behavioral functions, and some assist the subcortical activity of the emotion-directing amygdala and the pleasure-making reward center. In this manner the frontal insula enables the electric vibrations of feelings to influence much of mental life.

Empathy and Sympathy

The meaning of empathy overlaps the meaning of sympathy in current usage. But when someone defines empathy informally as "being on the same wave length" a clear difference in meaning with sympathy emerges. "Being on the same wave length" is metaphorically the same as resonating on the same frequency of a wave. And, according to the theory of loop circuits, that is what clusters of apical dendrites in the front insula are doing when a person has empathy with someone or with a group of individuals. Feeling sympathy with a person carries with it an understanding of the context of the feeling, and processing information about understanding things is presumed to take place in network circuits. Sympathy, then, is produced mainly by thinking while empathy is produced mainly by feeling. When people are bonded together by both a sharing of interests and a sharing of feelings, the bond is even stronger.

A remarkable observation made in human imaging studies is that the insula is not only activated by subjective emotions, but also when emotions are observed in another human being[9]. For example, in humans, the frontal insula is activated when a person experiences pain or a person observes pain in other people, or when someone tastes or sees other people taste pleasant or unpleasant food items. These data suggest a role for the frontal insula in mediating empathy, the ability to share the feelings of another individual. Humans who have difficulties in sensing their own emotional and bodily states, a condition called alexithymia, show less insula activation compared to most people when trying to assess their own feelings or the feelings of others[10]. These findings provide striking illustrations of the insula's role in linking the perception of social events with feelings.

A person who exhibits strong empathy for others is often described as having a "big heart." In view of the Loops Theory and data discussed in this book, it seems easier to imagine that strong empathy is related to a larger size of the insula in the brain than to a larger size of the physical heart in the chest.

The Insula and Social Affiliations

In a typical day, most people interact with other individuals, and when many individuals are involved, the interactions can be very complex. The neural structures of the brain apparently have evolved to support the many facets of social interactions. The frontal insula is prominent in social networking. In 2010, a review[11] of studies of socially relevant functions of the insula described the involvement of the frontal insula in empathy, compassion, fairness, and cooperation.

More recently, a 2018 study[12] examined the relationship between the frontal insula and social networking in two large samples of people, one group in New York City and the other group in Beijing, China. As a measure of social networking, the authors used the social network index (SNI) which summarizes each individual's network diversity, size, and complexity. An image of the frontal insula of each individual was obtained from their magnetic resonance image. Two features of the front insula correlated with the social network index: the measure of the volume of the frontal insula and the measure of the depth of the cortical valley in the frontal insula (see Figure 9.1). The volume of the amygdala (a structure connected with the insula which, as described earlier, orchestrates the many bodily responses during an emotion) also showed a correlation with the social network index. The authors concluded that the evidence from both New York and Beijing groups support the hypothesis that the frontal insula is an active contributor to our experiences of social interactions.

Individuals differ in their abilities to perceive their own feelings, which impacts their ability to infer the feelings of others. But whenever a particular occasion arouses feelings that are empathetically shared, a social bond is formed among these individuals. Strangers standing on a street corner who have just witnessed an automobile accident begin to notice each other and subsequently find it more easily to talk to each other. Singers in a chorus who have shared the same heights of feelings singing music feel closer to each other. Creating a strong social bond of empathy, according to the loops theory, involves the learning of new loops in not only the frontal insula but also in the areas that activate the insula, including the visual areas that process faces, and the areas that control the ways attention is directed to a face (see Figure 8.4).

Feelings and the Mysterious VEN: The Von Economo Neuron

Studies of the frontal insula and nearby frontal areas in large-brain mammals have revealed a neuron that is located within clusters of many pyramidal neurons. This large but slender neuron is named the Von Economo Neuron (VEN)[13] for the scientist who discovered it. Figure 9.2 (in the center and on the right side) shows examples of the VEN. On the left side of this figure is a pyramidal neuron for the purpose of making comparisons with the VEN. The right side of this figure shows cell bodies of VENs, which are highly magnified to show the large-diameter axons that leave the cell body.

VENs are not only found in the insula but also in the anterior cingulate area, an area of the frontal cortex[14], which, like the insula, participates in the flexible control of goal-directed activities. Some VENs have been observed in the attention areas above the eye (the orbitofrontal areas), discussed earlier as involved in attention to feelings. These findings led Allman[15] to suggest that these neurons produce social awareness.

It has been observed that VENs appear in the brains of highly social animals such as whales, dolphins. elephants, great apes and humans. The number of VENs found in the brains of humans varies greatly across different individuals, which may account for the wide differences among humans in sensitivity to their inner states and to the inner states of others.

Since VEN axons themselves are unusually large, and larger axons conduct pulses faster, Allman[15] in 2011 proposed that VENs could enable signals to be sent more quickly from the frontal insular hub to more distant frontal regions. In the brains of large social animals, fast communication by VENs would help an individual react faster and more effectively during quick changes in social interactions. Therefore the rapid communication by VENs to brain areas serving social actions confers a selective advantage to the members of a species that possesses these VENs.

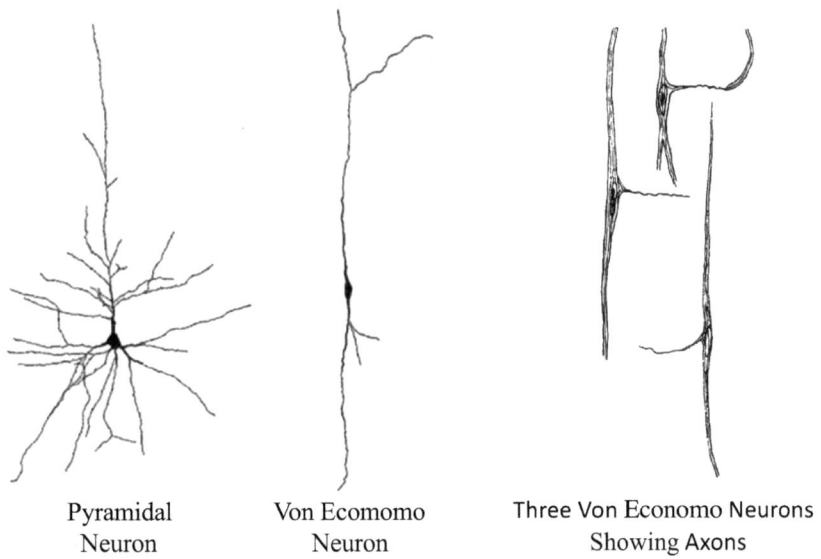

Pyramidal
Neuron

Von Ecomomo
Neuron

Three Von Economo Neurons
Showing Axons

Figure 9.2

The close proximity of a VEN to the apical dendrites of the pyramidal neurons which surround it suggests that the electric vibrations of the apical dendrites of these tightly packed neurons may directly affect the electric vibrations within the VEN. Figure 9.3 illustrates the close spacing of a VEN to surrounding pyramidal apical dendrites within a cluster of pyramidal neurons. (Note that, for purposes of illustration, a vertical VEN fiber in Figure 9.3 is drawn much thicker and much shorter than vertical VEN fibers shown in Figure 9.2.)

The direct interaction between closely spaced neurons is called ephaptic coupling, and this occurs when the electric field of the one neural fiber causes another fiber to vibrate at the same frequency and intensity. Ephaptic coupling is an alternative to the synapse as a way of passing electric activity from one neuron to another. The importance of ephaptic coupling to mental activity has yet to be determined but Loops Theory suggests a possible role for this means of excitation when neurons are packed together in close proximity.

A 2011 experiment[16] by Anastassiou, Perin, Markram, and Koch reported that ephaptic influences can occur at distances of at least 180 microns. Many apical dendrites of pyramidal neurons can crowd around a single VEN owing to the relative large size of the VEN, and even dendrites behind the first row of surrounding dendrites can fall within the 180 micron distance of ephaptic coupling. The cell bodies of VENs shown in Figure 9.2 contain an apical dendrite at the top and a similar dendrite at the bottom, and both resemble apical dendrites of pyramidal neurons. These two extended dendrites run parallel to the surrounding pyramidal apical dendrites for long distances within a cluster of apical dendrites. Separations between the VEN and its surrounding pyramidal apical dendrites are smaller than the approximately 50 micron (micrometer) diameter of a minicolumn that contains the apical dendrite bundle of about six fibers[17].

Ephaptic coupling is the direct interaction between closely spaced neurons that occurs when the electric field of one neural fiber causes

Von Economo Neuron (VEN) Inside
A Cluster of Apical Dendrites

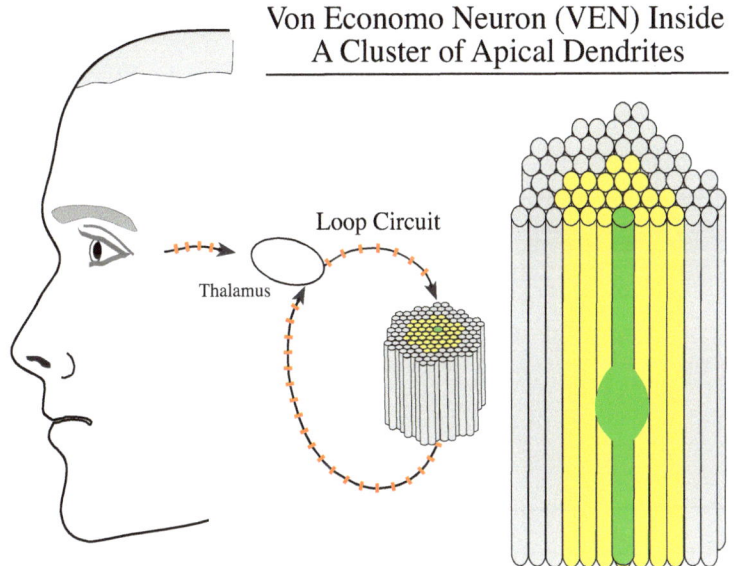

Thalamus

Loop Circuit

Figure 9.3

the electric field of another fiber to vibrate electrically with the same frequency. The average distance between adjacent apical dendrites within a bundle is no more than 30 microns[17], which is well below the approximately 180 micron limit reported for electric field interactions between adjacent neurons in the 2011 (Anastasslou et al) study[16].

In the normal human brain the total number of VENs is counted in the thousands, while the number of pyramidal apical dendrites in which the VENs are embedded is counted in the millions. When a thousand VENs are scattered across a million pyramidal neurons, the VEN typically finds itself alone among a crowd of pyramidal neurons. Thus, the VEN is usually a solitary contributor to the activity of a cluster of other (pyramidal) neurons. When pulses from this lonely fiber, along with pulses from its crowd of surrounding neurons, arrive at another cortical area, what do the VEN pulses do at the target area that is different from what the surrounding pyramidal pulses do? It seems likely that the pulses of the VEN reach the target area sooner than the other pulses in the cluster of fibers, owing to their larger size. But is that the only processing advantage that the VEN provides? Additional research is needed to answer this question. Meanwhile, there is reason for optimism in the prospect of forming new VENs by learning experiences because of the existing evidence for the learning of new apical dendrites of pyramidal neurons described in Chapter 7. Adding a new VEN to a cluster of pyramidal apical dendrites could come about in the same way that a new pyramidal neuron is added to an existing bundle of pyramidal neurons: A brief burst of pulses from a thalamic axon fiber raises the voltage at a synapse located at the top of the VEN as it does to a synapse at the top of the apical dendrite.

Research into the detailed operations of these intriguing VENs is young, but more studies are welcomed by a wide range of cognitive scientists because most of these neurons are located in the frontal areas that produce feelings and social networking.

Chapter 10

Being on the Same Wavelength

Do you remember an awkward moment when you had just been introduced to someone and you were straining to find something that you both knew about, something that could put you on the same wavelength for some conversation?

Being on the same wavelength with someone means to share similar opinions or feelings about something, and this sharing has become so important to us that our language has picked up many ways of saying the same thing. Examples are: *being on the same page, seeing eye to eye, being of one mind, in tune with, in sync, to click with*. Getting on the same wavelength is the first step toward forming successful relationships with friends, neighbors, professional colleagues and clients. In short, it smooths the paths of social networking.

The key to connecting with each other socially is communication, whether by human language or by the gestures of ants or by the simple on-off electric signaling of neurons. But exchanging words, gestures, or electric signals, is only one part of communication. This book highlights another important part of the communication process which is the timing of the signals as they are sent and received. In other words, communication between individuals involves not only the information in the message, but also how the message is sent, in particular the time intervals between the signals that make up the message. It turns out that this is also true for communication between neurons within the nervous system.

One way to illustrate the importance of the timings between signals is trying to understand the following vocal sounds: "Ohwah tahgoo siam." Most people cannot understand this series of sounds the first several times that they hear them. But they can easily understand these sounds if the time interval between each syllable is made almost the same, so that they hear: "Oh what a goose I am."

When we want to make sure that a listener understands exactly what we are saying, we speak the words slowly so that we can make the intervals between them about the same to help make the sound of each word clear. In other words, communication involves not only the information in the message, but also how the message is sent, in particular the time intervals between the signals that make up the message.

The simplest way to control the moment that a sound signal is sent out is to put the signals on a specific wavelength or frequency, often called a carrier frequency. This happens when we use small handheld devices and the larger devices of computers, TVs, and radios. It is important to understand that frequency and wavelength are interchangeable measurments when transmitting waves through the same material, such as air, water, or cortical tissue. If we know the frequency of a wave, we can calculate its wave length simply by dividing 1 by the frequency, and vice versa.[1]

Waves breaking on a beach can be measured by the distance between their wave peaks, which is their wavelength, or they can be measured by the number of wave peaks arriving per second, which is their frequency. When we listen to small waves lapping on a shore line, we are more aware of the frequency of waves, and when we look at large waves crashing on a beach, we are more aware of the wavelength of waves.

As described earlier, we choose a particular wavelength (or frequency) when we tune a radio or TV to a particular broadcasting station, and pilots in the air connect with other pilots by tuning their radios to a shared frequency or wavelength. In order for a computer to ensure successful communication of signals in its network of wires and computing devices all of the computations (outputs) that are taking place in different locations must take place at exactly the same time. Therefore, the time intervals between the computer signals (pulse or no-pulse) in different messages must all match so that when the outputs of these separate computations eventually come together at a new location, each ordered pulse or space in the separate messages will make contact at precisely the same time.

Synchronizing the many operations of a computer is like getting a group of soldiers to march in time, and like getting a group of musicians to play their notes in time. Keeping time needs a steady signal to assure that each interval of time between a step or a note is precisely the same. In music, a steady beat is usually maintained internally by a performer, or expressed externally by tapping a foot or by watching the arm movements of a conductor. A computer synchronizes its operations by means of a system clock (for example, a small quartz crystal) that is located on the central motherboard of the computer and resonates at 32,768 cycles per second (when an electric current is fed to it). Getting computer devices to operate on the same wavelength or frequency is an easy problem to solve: just attach an external clock device that sends out signals that are equally spaced in time. But getting neurons to operate on the same wavelength/frequency has turned out to be a very difficult problem, mainly because, unlike the reliable transmission of electric pulses across junctions of wires, the transmission of electric pulses across synaptic junctions of most neurons randomly disturbs the timing of the pulses. Most synapses operate electro-chemically, and at this molecular level quasi-random fluctuations are always present.

So, how does the brain produce the kind of steady signals needed to precisely synchronize the steps of information processing when these steps are occurring at different locations of a neural network?

Getting Neurons to Send Pulses At the Same Frequency (Wave Length) With Vibrations of the Apical Dendrite: A Neural Clock

It turns out that the long apical dendrite in a loop circuit can act as a surprisingly precise clock. The pyramidal neuron that contains the apical dendrite can send out a very steady series of pulses to synchronize the workings of other neurons which enables those neurons to talk to each other on the same frequency/wavelength.

Another benefit of timing neural activity with a loop circuit is the ability of a loop to send out pulses at *any* frequency within the range of a neuron's output, rather than setting the clock pulses at only one frequency, as is the case for a network in the typical computer. We already know that the range of firing rates of a neural fiber is 1 Hz to 1000 Hz (based on the minimum time of one millisecond for the axon fiber to recover from a spike), but usually single spikes (regular firing) and bursts (burst firing) occur within the range of 1 Hz to 100 Hz, while the rate of spikes within a burst is believed to be within the range of about 100 to 700 Hz[2].

The frequency of pulses within a loop circuit can be quickly modified by changing the frequency of pulses in the long vertical axons of layer 6 pyramidal neurons (see the diagram of a minicolumn in Figure 10.1) which travel upward toward the cortical surface along the outside of the layer 5 apical dendrite membrane. Here, for present purposes, the vertical lines that arise from layer 6 neurons represent axons instead of apical dendrites. Figure 10.2 shows these long vertical axons of layer 6 pyramidal neurons that make synaptic contacts with vertical apical dendrites of layer 5 neurons in Figure 10.2B, and Figure 10.2A shows the axons from thalamic neurons that terminate on layer 4 stellate neurons whose locations are distributed haphazardly[3]. The long vertical axons

The Cortical Minicolumn

Layers

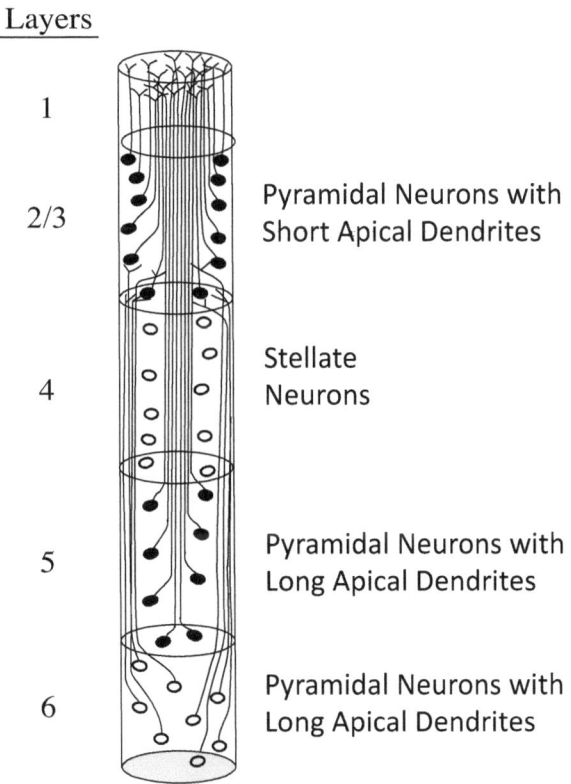

1

2/3   Pyramidal Neurons with
       Short Apical Dendrites

4   Stellate
       Neurons

5   Pyramidal Neurons with
       Long Apical Dendrites

6   Pyramidal Neurons with
       Long Apical Dendrites

Figure 10.1

Axons of Layer 6 Pyramidal Neurons that Terminate on Layer 4 Stellate Neurons (A), and Contact the Many Spines Of a Layer 5 Apical Dendrite (B)

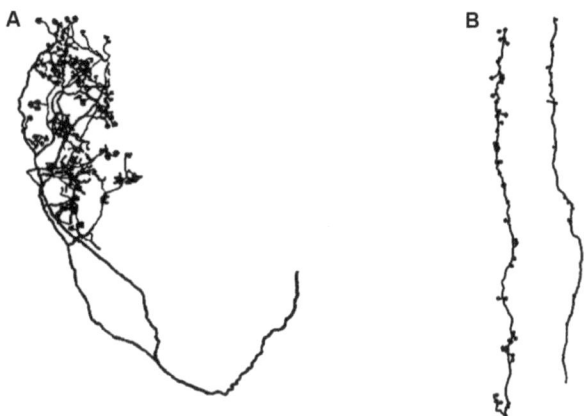

Figure 10.2

have the appearance of vines that attach themselves to a wall for support as they grow. The contacts with the wall correspond to the many synapses by which the layer 6 axons regulate the frequency of vibrations along the dendritic shaft of the apical dendrite of a pyramidal layer 5 neuron.

Layer 6 pyramidal neurons, like those of layer 5, are part of loop circuits and their mode of operation keeps pulses moving around the loop at a very steady rate. The pulse frequency of the layer 6 loop circuit is set by fibers originating in the frontal cortex, where voluntary choices are made (revisit Figure 6.6). Although a pyramidal neuron of layer 5 can produce different levels of attention by varying the number of spikes in a burst (see Figure 6.1), a layer 6 pyramidal neuron sets its frequency with regular firings of single pulses. Layer 6 pyramidal neurons rarely show burst-firing[4,5].

Therefore, in the figures of this book the activity levels of layer 6 neurons are colored yellow (for single-pulse activity), while the activity levels of level 5 neurons are also colored orange or red (for small or large bursts of pulses) to indicate low or high levels of attention (see Figure 6.2). The regulatory frequency of the pyramidal neuron of layer 6 is assumed to be initially set and then maintained by a control circuit in the frontal lobe.

The long axons of layer 6 pyramidal neurons contact not only the apical dendrites of layer 5 and 6 pyramidal neurons, but they also contact the short layer 2 or 3 pyramidal neurons within a column of neurons (each column contains about 100 minicolumns). They do this by sending pulses along axon fibers that run vertically along the outside of the apical dendrites in such a way that the axon fibers contact the hundreds of synapses that dot the outside of an apical dendrite. Therefore axons of layer 6 pyramidal neurons typically tune all of the apical dendrites, long and short, within a column of 100 minicolumns to a common frequency.

A major benefit of setting the resonating frequencies of so many apical dendrites in a column to the same wavelength (or frequency) is that these neurons can then dominate mental activity. The resonating of the apical dendrites maintains these anticipations up to the moment that the anticipated event occurs or when we make the anticipated response. The action of setting and sustaining the resonating frequency of large numbers of apical dendrites can be illustrated by a conductor of an orchestra. The conductor selects the tempo and insures that the timing of the beats is maintained by moving his or her arms. In most of the music heard today, a note is begun and ended at a specific time that is determined by the rhythmic pulse-beat of the tempo with which a piece of music is played. Every player in the group must "feel the beat" to make sounds that are synchronized in tempo.

In a minicolumn of neurons, the long apical dendrite of the layer 6 neuron is the "conductor" who is responsible for making the pulses in loop circuits occur at a particular frequency, thereby maintaining the same time interval between each pulse. In the field of music, the shortest conductor can keep a beat as well as the tallest conductor, but in the field of neuroscience the longer the apical dendrite the more precise the timing of the pulse (beat).

Evidence that the Apical Dendrite Can Fine-Tune Itself

Evidence that apical dendrites fine-tune themselves first appeared in a 2011 article by Ray Kasevich and myself[6,7]. This article describes a mathematical model and a simulation of what happens in an apical dendrite when the dendrite receives a steady series of electric pulses in its loop circuit. The electric pulses entering the top of the apical dendrite produce surges of current whose intensity (voltage) lies below the level that produces a spike in an axon. Because of the importance of this distinction between the low intensities of electric activity in the apical dendrite and the relatively high intensities of pulses in axons, the terms surges and spikes, respectively, are used.

We modeled the apical dendrite as a series of 7 compartments, of which 6 represented the shaft of the apical dendrite, and then we looked for an equation that describes the way that electric activity at the beginning of one compartment changes to produce the electric activity at the beginning of the next compartment. By modeling a series of compartments instead of the whole apical dendrite it is possible to write an equation that describes the electric effect of moving surges along the apical dendrite upon the frequency of its electric vibrations.

The electric activity in a neuron depends upon many factors (parameters), including the length of the apical dendrite, the width of the membrane and core, and the many electrical properties that govern the passage of electric current along an apical dendrite. It was soon clear to us that the equation that expressed the operation of all these factors while surges of current moved down the apical dendrite would be very complex. Fortunately, Ray, who is an electrical physicist, soon found a book by Delogne[7] that contained the equation we needed.

Of all the parameters in the Delogne equation, the rate of potassium outflow through the many channels in the membrane is the only component of the equation that changes from compartment to compartment. This is important because the rate of outward potassium flow is presumed to directly affect the momentary frequency of surges in a compartment.

The foregoing considerations led me to write a simple difference equation (a differential equation written in discrete form instead of in continuous form) for the change in outward potassium flow as a function of the number of cycles around the loop circuit instead of the number of compartments[8]. This linear difference equation was easily solved[9,10], and the many physiological parameter values involved in energy transfer from one compartment to the next were available from recent publications.

The results of the simulation showed resonance curves (vibration curves) for each of the peak frequencies of 20, 40, 60, and 80 Hz and the 60Hz curves are in Figure 10.3. The shapes of the frequency profiles, which start as a flat horizontal line, begin to resemble a mountain with a peak that grows sharper and sharper with every loop traversed by the surges of current along the apical dendrite. The peak is always located near the average frequency of pulses that the axons of the layer 6 neuron axons deliver to the synapses on the apical dendrite at hundreds of locations along its shaft (see Figure 10.2 earlier in this chapter and the description of the way the layer 6 axons contact the many synapses along a layer 5 apical dendrite).

At the beginning of the looping activity, the durations of the time interval between current surges were not equal but changed duration randomly from one pair of pulses to the next pair. This high variability in duration is indicted by the wide width of the frequency profile which was initially flat (note that, for each profile curve, the height of the curve at a specific frequency represents the percentage of times that frequency is observed). After 6 to 8 cycles through 6 compartments of the apical dendrite shaft, these intervals became almost equal, as indicated by the narrow width of the frequency profiles (when the profile is almost a vertical line, all the frequencies are crowded around the same peak frequency value, which indicates that the time between each pair of pulses is exactly the same). In other words, the apical dendrite membrane acted on the passing pulses in a manner that made the pulse movements more and more steady, and eventually, the time between surges approached the steadiness of the pulses of the quartz crystal that serves as a clock for timing the computations in a computer.

The finding that the movement of pulse surges along the apical dendrite produces a sharp mountain-like peak in the frequency profile and that the frequency of this peak matches the regulating frequency of the pulses in the axon of a pyramidal neuron of layer 6 can be more simply described as *tuning* the apical dendrite to vibrate at the peak frequency value. The additional finding that the observed frequencies crowd closer to the peak frequency with every pass around the loop (making the intervals between pulses more similar) can be more simply described as *fine-tuning* the apical dendrite.

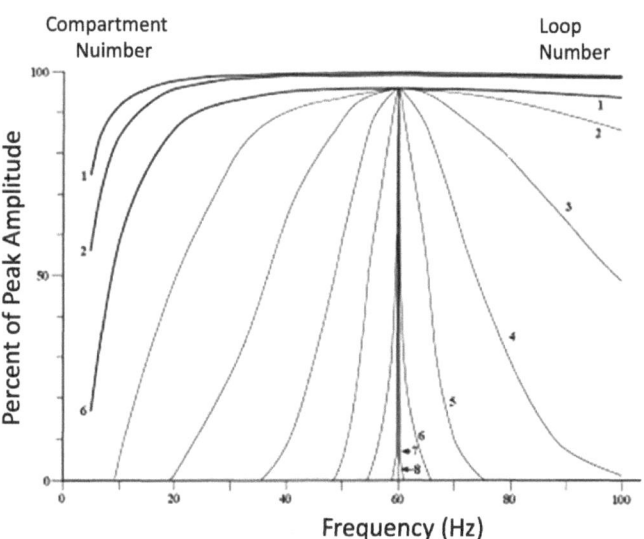

Figure 10.3

The level of fine-tuning achieved by an apical dendrite depends on how long it is and how on how many times that electric current flows through the apical dendrite. Every pass through the loop adds neural noise produced by the synapses at the thalamus and at the top of the apical dendrite. Longer apical dendrites contain more compartments, and so a string of pulses can receive more fine tuning before passing through synapses in the loop circuit. Very short apical dendrites, as found in mice, have only a few compartments, and the amount of refinement from one pass through the apical dendrite may be canceled by the flattening effect of synaptic noise in the loop circuit. As a result, the apical dendrite may give little or no benefit to the processing in the network neurons of the mice.

In contrast, the long length of the apical dendrite may have reached a limit in the human, because present simulations of a 6-compartment model of the apical dendrites show that only a relatively few cycles of pulses around the apical dendrite loop may be sufficient to produce a resonance curve that is almost a vertical line, indicating that the variability of pulse intervals has been reduced virtually to zero (see Figure 10.3).

In general terminology, the frequency profile of apical dendrite processing may be called the resonance profile (or resonance curve) of the apical dendrite activity, following the conventional use of the term *resonance* in the field of physics. The frequency at the peak of the profile is called the resonant frequency, regardless of whether the profile is narrow or wide.

An active apical dendrite continuously influences activities in many circuits of the brain, and therefore it is important for the apical dendrite to maintain a steady output of pulses (a sharp resonance profile). However, keeping a long apical dendrite membrane resonating at very narrow band of frequencies is a "high-maintenance" job that involves the membrane of the entire shaft of the apical dendrite, as hundreds of synapses continually squirt small groups of sodium ions into it and hundreds of channels continually pass small groups of potassium ions out of it. This prolonged activity of the apical dendrite contrasts with the relatively brief activity in an axon when a small section of an axon produces its electric spike.

Up to this point, this chapter has focused on the way that the apical dendrite can operate as a timer of electrical changes in the cortical networks of the brain. This timing operation was described by the present mathematical model of apical dendrite activity, developed by Ray Kasevich and myself, which shows how pulse surges passing along the apical dendrite can be tuned to any frequency within the range of a neuron, like a radio or TV set can be tuned to any particular frequency/wavelength within their ranges. Our simulation experiment reported in a 2011 article[6] shows that the apical dendrite can also be fine-tuned to produce pulses at very precise time intervals, which is necessary to make sure that the outputs of all computations are performed at virtually the same time, as they are in computers.

One of the major benefits of being able to tune neurons by using the vibrations of the apical dendrite is that the apical dendrite can easily be tuned to any frequency within its range (usually between 0 and about 100 Hz), while the typical computer clock runs at only one frequency. For example, the frequency of the apical dendrite that controls the action plan for parking the car can run at a different frequency than the apical dendrite that controls the action plan for stopping at a red light, or the action plan for passing another car on a highway. Hence, choosing the next thing to do by the brain may be greatly simplified by choosing a particular frequency to dominate the current operations of cortical circuits. Also, after choosing a particular action plan by choosing a frequency, we can narrow down what to do next by using attention to raise the activation of a particular response within that cluster (revisit Figure 6.6). So, the act of shifting from one of these clusters to another cluster can also be made quickly by selecting a frequency which, in turn, selects the circuit that runs on that frequency. The brain does this when our thinking shifts from topic to topic, such as when we consider what we might do for fun next weekend and we jump from possibility to possibility.

Application of the Loops Theory to the Formation and Operation Of a Context in Mental Activity

Getting dressed in the morning involves doing many things that usually take time. Even choosing the right clothes for the day can take up a lot of time when one's wardrobe provides many options. The number of possible decisions about what to do in the next moment has already been drastically reduced by having chosen the context of getting dressed.

Let us consider how the circuits that serve getting dressed might be involved in this example. The "getting dressed" circuits are organized into a larger group of circuits that correspond to a context or topic (the name of the context). The neural basis for this organization is a specific loop circuit that contains a long apical dendrite, as illustrated in Figure 10.4. In this figure, the group of neural circuits that make up a context are colored yellow.

The neural activity for getting dressed is produced by the apical dendrite (colored yellow) within a loop circuit, which controls the frequency of vibrations in the connected network circuit (colored blue). The many (yellow-coded) network circuits that the loop circuit activates are spread out on each side of the location of the loop circuit. The red network and loop circuits represent elevated attention while searching for a very specific choice of clothes such as which shirt to wear. The ribbon-like view of the network sheet in Figure 10.4 is from the inside of the brain when the brain is divided in half vertically at the center.

If one observes the whole brain from the outside as in Figure 10.5 then the network sheet resembles a broad surface like the roof of an arena. Near the center of this surface are the tips at the tops of the loop circuits (colored yellow) representing the long apical dendrites, which connect with many short apical dendrites that represent the network neurons that serve the currently active context.

Network Circuits of Context and Attention
Selected by Loop Circuits

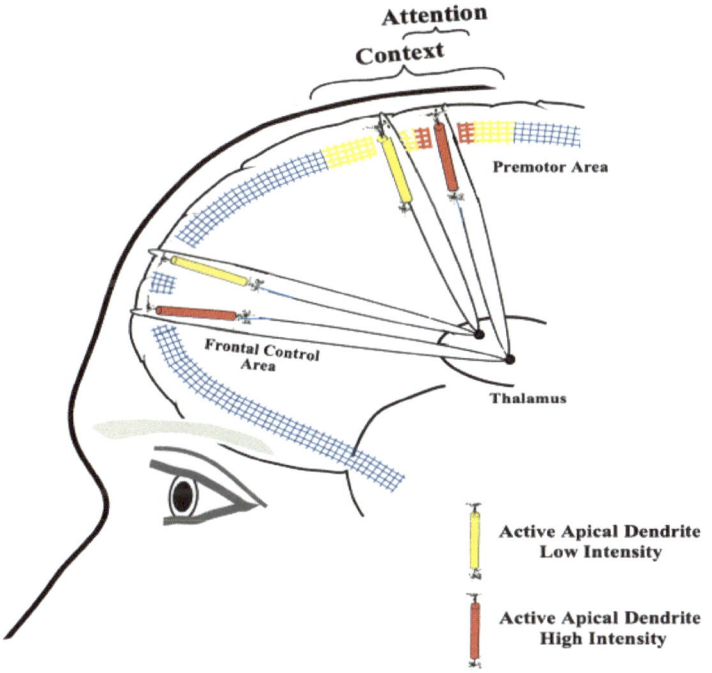

Figure 10.4

Network Circuits Representing a Context and
An Attended Part of that Context

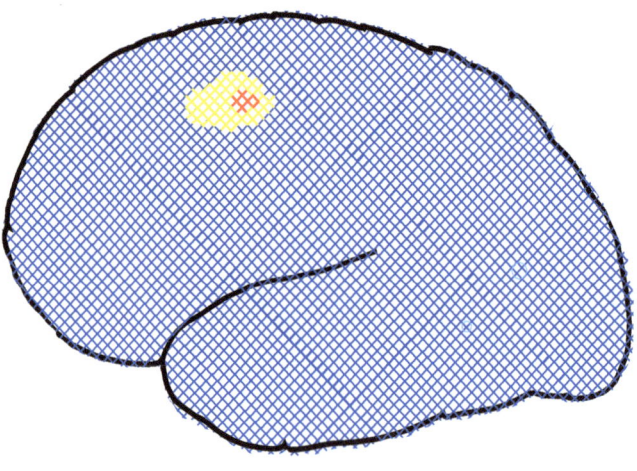

Figure 10.5

Within this group of active context neurons is a smaller group of loop circuit tips (colored red) which have been activated by attention. Attentional activation is usually more narrowly focused than contextual activation, and this nested feature depicts the ability of attention to pinpoint the location of small group of network circuits within the larger group of circuits of a context. For example, a loop circuit in the frontal lobe (colored yellow) that controls the general contextual topic of getting dressed activates a long pyramidal neuron in layer 6 (colored yellow in a loop circuit), which is located in a minicolumn of the cortex (colored yellow), and a frontal area (colored red) that provides the attentional activation of choosing a green shirt activates a long pyramidal neuron in layer 5 (colored red) in the cortical sheet. Thus, pyramidal neurons in layer 5 become active when a specific part or aspect of a context receives attention.

The difference in function between the long apical dendrites of pyramidal neurons in layer 5 and layer 6 is expressed in the mode of firing of these neurons. Layer 6 pyramidal neurons show regular firing of single pulses and seldom show burst firing[3,4], while layer 5 pyramidal neurons can show either regular firing, or burst firing in groups of 2 to 7 spikes (see Figure 6.1).

The use of a yellow code to represent regular firing within a loop circuit may be confusing in the case of selecting a context of network circuits, because other contexts also have yellow-coded network circuits. How does a particular control circuit activate neurons that lie only within the context of momentary interest without involving neurons of other contexts?

According to the present theory, the selection of a particular context in the frontal cortical area is produced by choosing a specific frequency for the apical dendrite loop that makes contact in the thalamus with the loop that selects the circuit of the momentary context (see Figure 10.4), where a small section of the blue coded network circuitry is colored yellow). The circuits that produce the context are also shown as a yellow circle in Figure 10.5, where the large sheet of network circuits is viewed from outside of the whole brain.

After processing has taken place in the circuits that serve the context, axon outputs are sent to muscle groups that execute overt actions. The pulse patterns carried by these axon outputs are produced by network neurons whose membranes vibrate at thee same frequency as the originating apical dendrites of the frontal control circuits. (How membranes of neurons are made to vibrate while the neurons process pulse information will be described in the next section of this chapter). In other words, the neurons that participate in the contextual operations, beginning with the frontal control loops and ending at the neurons that produce muscle outputs all vibrate at the same frequency. Having the same membrane vibration frequency for all neurons serving a particular context also protects the neural operations from interference by neural events in circuits of other contexts that use other membrane frequencies.

The small group of red-coded circuits within the (yellow-coded) contextual circuits of Figures 10.4 and 10.5 represent the neurons whose firings are momentarily intensified by shifting from single-firing to burst firing. The selection of these attentional neurons parallels the selection of the context neurons: First, circuits in the frontal area of voluntary control select loop circuits of a particular frequency of vibration, and these loop circuits connect in the thalamus with loop circuits that contact the red-coded contextual circuits within the large network sheet. A familiar illustrative example in the context of getting dressed in the morning is deciding what shoes to wear.

The diagram in Figure 10.4 shows the area of frontal control that selects a group of context circuits and a group of attention circuits in the cortical network. The route of each control-to-network circuit is made of two loops which are connected in the thalamus. When the momentary context is shifted from one group of network circuits to another group (e.g., shifting from driving to parking, or from getting dressed to eating breakfast), the brain shifts activation from one control loop to another control loop. Each new control loop then activates its connected loop in the thalamus that activates a group of network circuits that represents an action plan.

The Bridges that Connect Loop Circuits to Network Circuits

Up to this point in this chapter we have used the metaphor of being on the same wavelength to describe how two network circuits can communicate with each other and carry out the processing of information being sent between them. To put two network circuits on the same wave length requires some other neural structure to control the electric vibrations of the membranes of the two neurons. Earlier sections of this chapter described in general terms how the loop circuit could provide this kind of influence on the network circuits, but details of the connections between the loop circuit and the network circuits were not spelled out. These details are described here after providing some background.

A diagram of network and loop circuits in the brain was shown earlier in Figure 5.2. In this figure, the blue ribbon represents the interlacing of relatively small network circuits within the thin sheet of neurons that spreads across the brain, and it lies beneath the outer surface of the brain, while loop circuits are represented by black lines. Only a cross-section of the thin sheet of neurons is shown in Figure 5.2.

The network sheet shown in Figure 5.2 is penetrated by the tips of the loop circuits of apical dendrites (also see Figure 10.5), which indicates that each loop circuit connects with a small group of network circuits that lie near the point of contact with the network sheet. Figure 5.2 shows that network circuits can also be contacted by a direct route from the thalamus that does not involve the loop circuit. For example, people in the background of the person we are attending to are registered in our brains without the participation of a cortical loop of attention.

If loops and networks work in very different ways and produce very different outputs, then how can they be made to influence each other at the point where a loop connects with the network? What kind of bridge between electric vibrations and pulses would allow a vibration to interact with the processing of pulses?

One solution, suggested by looking at the available neural hardware, is to find a neuron that engages in both electric vibrations and pulse processing, which at first seems unlikely, given what is known about neurons. However, in the context of Loops Theory, there is such a neuron and that neuron is the short pyramidal neuron, the neuron that contains the short apical dendrite (revisit Figure 3.2). This neuron is located in layers 2 and 3 of the cortex (see Figures 10.1 and 10.6). Two of these neurons are shown in Figure 10.6. Each apical dendrite of these neurons receives activation from the big loop of the long pyramidal neuron and transfers this activity to its cell body. In effect, the apical dendrite serves as a "bridge" for conveying vibrational activity from the long pyramidal neuron to the cell body of the short pyramidal neuron. The very small distance between the cell body of a layer 2 neuron and its axon synapse makes observation of the short shaft of the layer 2 pyramidal neuron difficult to observe in microphotographs. Therefore for clarity in the drawing of Figure 10.6, the thickness of the network sheet (colored blue) is made thin when it actually should be thick enough to include the cell bodies and apical dendrites of the neurons of layers 2 and 3.

The important point here is that short pyramidal neurons enable the vibrating loop circuit to connect with the network circuits of the cortex. The apical dendrite of the short pyramidal neuron resembles a bridge that serves as a border between two adjacent European countries. One country represents loop circuits and the other country represents network circuits. The upper end of the apical dendrite connects with the loop country, and the lower end of the apical dendrite connects with the network country. When the loop country activates the apical dendrite it vibrates electrically and its vibrations spread across the bridge and make the cell body and basal dendrites

Loop Circuit Connects to Network Circuits Across Bridges of Short Apical Dendrites

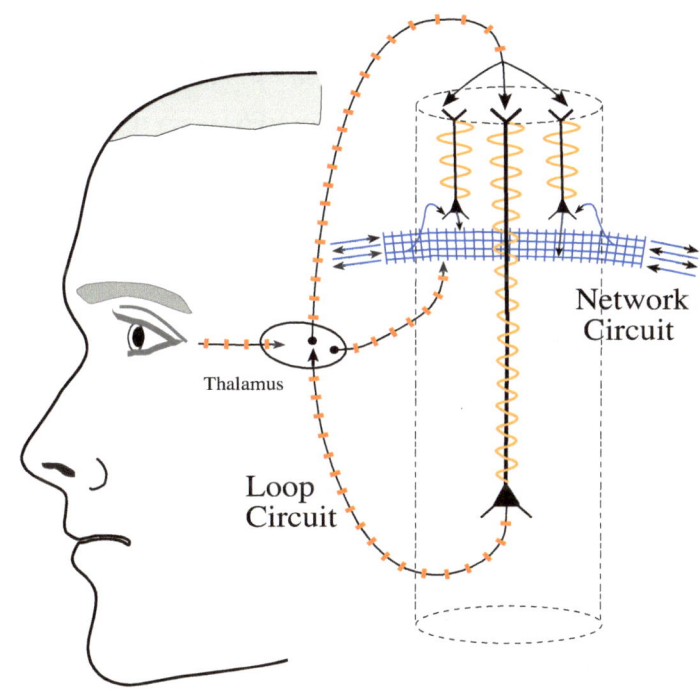

Figure 10.6

vibrate with the same frequency. As a result, both countries now vibrate with the same frequency

No pulse information is carried across the bridge by the spreading vibration because the loop country has no information to transmit. Therefore the only outcome of activity on the bridge is the spread of a vibration[11] from the loop country to the network country. The cell body and the basal dendrites of the network country will continue to vibrate as long as the bridge neuron (the short pyramidal neuron) is active. At the same time, electric vibrations at the same frequency are spreading across bridges in the many short pyramidal neurons in same minicolumn (see Figure 10.1) because the big loop is also connected to the other short pyramidal neurons. Figure 10.6 shows the big loop's connection with two of these bridge neurons, but typically a long pyramidal in layer 6 is connected via a loop circuit to many short pyramidal neurons within its minicolumn, (and also within the other minicolumns that make up a column). As a result, all of the short pyramidal neurons in layers 2 and 3 of a column of 100 minicolumns can cause a very large network of surrounding neurons to vibrate at the same frequency.

When all the neurons in a network vibrate at the same frequency, then any of these neurons can communicate with any other neuron that connects to that network. This conclusion can be expressed by the following hypothesis:

> *A neuron will accept a series of pulses from another neuron if and only if their membranes vibrate at the same frequency and are in phase.*

This hypothesis, which here is derived from the assumptions of the Loops Theory, was proposed and supported by evidence in a 2015 study by Fries[14].

A great deal of research over the past 30 years has investigated the ways that two neurons can be made to fire together. Called "neural binding," the implications of this notion have captured the interests not only of neuroscientists, but also of psychologists and philosophers. Psychologists attempted to discover how the perception of red color and square shape are combined to produce the perception of a red square, and philosophers wondered how the experience of color and the experience of shape become unified in a conscious experience of an object that combines them.

The idea of neural binding of neurons has been expanded to the binding of large groups of neurons that produce cognition. The 2015 article by Fries[14] proposed that synchronization at gamma-band frequencies (30-90 Hz) affects communication between neuronal groups and changes in synchronization can flexibly alter the pattern of communications among the neurons of these groups.

The Role of Membrane Vibrations
in the Transmission of Pulses Between Neurons

The matching of frequencies between two communicating neurons in a network goes to the root of the claim, made by this book, that resonating neurons in loop circuits are necessary for the computer-like information processing in the network circuits of the brain. Being connected to the same loop circuit assures that all the neurons that are to communicate with each other will vibrate at the same frequency.

It should be emphasized that the loop circuit does not send pulses of information across the neural bridge but instead it makes the bridge resonate at a particular frequency; and this resonating frequency is passed along to the membranes of the cell body and basal dendrites of the short pyramidal neuron that contains the bridge. As a consequence, the cell body and the basal dendrites will continue to resonate if the bridge of the short apical dendrite keeps resonating. The sustaining of resonating in the short apical dendrite is made possible by the continued activity of the long apical dendrite in the large loop circuit. Therefore, the usual mode of activation of the loop circuit and its apical dendrite produces prolonged periods of resonating while the attached network neurons carry out their work of processing streams of information.

In order to visualize what is happening within a network neuron (the lower part of a short pyramidal neuron) when a series of spikes arrives at a synapse, Figures 10.7 and 10.8 show illustrative diagrams of the transmission of a series of pulses from one to another neuron. These figures show a short pyramidal neuron (a bridge neuron) containing spikes on the two input axons and spikes on the output axon. The insides of two horizontal dendrites carry trains of surges that result from the contact of input spikes on the two input axons.

Figure 10.8 expands the bottom (network) portion of Figure 10.7 to show the vibrations of the membrane that surrounds all parts of the short pyramidal neuron except the axon. The important things to observe in Figure 10.8 are: (1) the very top of the image corresponds to the junction that joins the bottom of the short apical dendrite to the top of the cell body of the neuron, and shown in this region are the vibrations of the membrane (grey arrow) and vibrations within the apical dendrite (blue arrow); (2) the vibrations of the membranes of the basal dendrites (diagrammed here in the horizontal membranes) are indicated by four red arrows; (3) the two input axons (axons from other neurons), contain spike trains, but only one (green arrow) has spikes that match the peaks of the resonating membrane.;(4) the other input axon, indicated by the purple arrow, contains spike trains that are not synchronous in timing with the peaks of the resonating membrane, and therefore there is no "match" and so no synapse is activated; (5) finally, this diagram implies that the axon output of this short pyramidal neuron may generate spike trains (orange arrow) which may or may not match the vibration frequency of another neuron's dendrite membrane. Thus, Figure 10.8 describes how an input of pulse trains will be accepted by a neuron if and only if the input spikes fit the peaks of the neuron's membrane vibrations.

Connecting to the Short Apical Dendrite

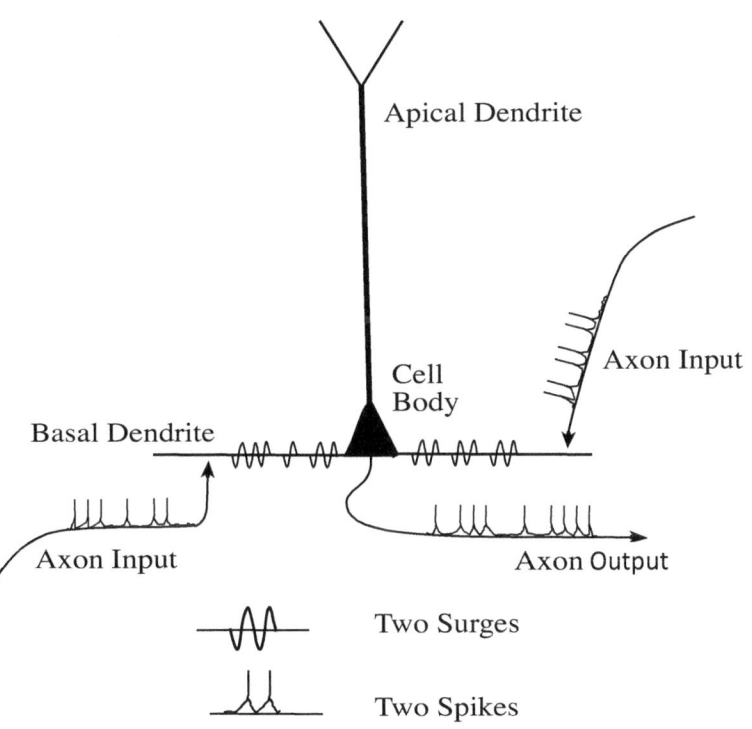

Figure 10.7

The Short Pyramidal Neuron:

The Timing of Spikes in the Input Axon
Must Match the Timing Of Vibrations
In the Membrane of the Neuron To
Be Accepted at a Synapse

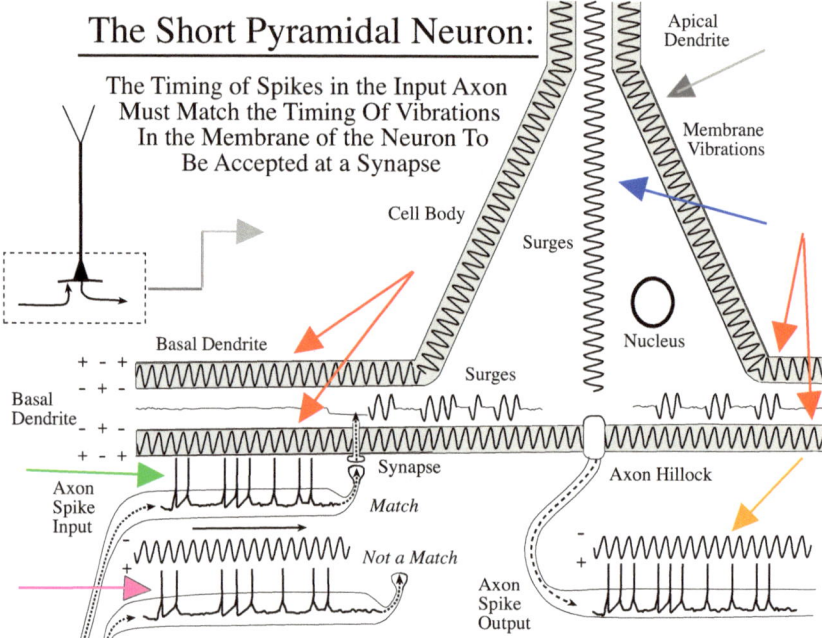

Figure 10.8

When we observe the pattern of spike trains in the input and output axons we note that there is no vibrating membrane surrounding the axon. However, the axon hillock, which is the part of the membrane of the neuron that discharges into its axon, does vibrate. Therefore, the pulses sent into the axon at the axon hillock will coincide with the peaks of the neuron's membrane vibrations. Since the transmission of pulse trains over the usual lengths of axons does not involve significant amounts of electric noise, the pattern of pulses that arrive at the end of the axon will have the same pattern as the pulses produced by the axon hillock at the cell body.

In the upper left part of this figure there is a small drawing of the short pyramidal neuron, and the rest of Figure 10.8 is devoted to showing an expanded view of the lower part of this neuron. A more detailed and technical description of membrane activity during neural transmission is provided in the footnote to this diagram[13].

This chapter is about the importance of timing in the communication of neurons with each other. A computer regulates the timing and speed of all of its functions by means of an external clock, but the brain regulates these things by loop circuits that contain apical dendrites. Like the electric pulses produced by a computer clock, the pulses produced by an apical dendrite must be precisely timed if their purpose is to keep the intervals between pulses the same. In terms of wave vibrations. the purpose is to keep the peak-to-peak distances of a wave the same.

In summary, a computer clock maintains a steady output of pulses by means of a quartz crystal, and a neural clock maintains a steady output of pulses by an apical dendrite that fine tunes itself to produce a steady output. This chapter gave a brief description of how the apical dendrite fine-tunes itself as pulses in its loop circuit make surges of current pass through it multiple times.

In order for a vibration in a loop circuit to produce the same vibration in a neuron of a network circuit the two neurons must contact each other in a special way. According to the Loops Theory of this book, the way vibrations of a long pyramidal neuron contact pulses in a network neuron takes place *within* a short pyramidal neuron. The upper part of a short pyramidal neuron is an apical dendrite, which receives its vibrations from a loop neuron that contains a long pyramidal neuron, and the lower part of a short pyramidal neuron which contains the cell body axon and basal dendrite, which are parts of a network neuron.

What happens within the short pyramidal neuron when a loop neuron meets a network neuron is that the vibration in the apical dendrite of the upper part spreads to the cell body and the basal dendrites of the lower part of the short pyramidal neuron, as if the apical dendrite acts as a bridge between the upper and lower parts. When other short pyramidal neurons that are connected to the same loop circuit are also active, they cause many network neurons to vibrate at the same frequency. The neurons in all of these circuits will now vibrate at the same frequency.

When two neurons share the same frequency of vibration, it is the vibration of their membranes that makes possible the transfer of pulse messages to each other. A diagram (Figure 10.8) of the vibrating membranes of the two neurons is provided as an assistance to understanding this way that two neurons communicate.

Chapter 11

Consciousness

Consciousness is customarily described as a state or a condition of the mind. In past chapters of this book we have considered states of mind, such as attention and feelings, in terms of the kind of neural circuits that give rise to them. It is much easier to regard these states, and states in general, as arising from the steady outputs of loop circuits rather than from network circuits. Of all the mental states studied, the one that is most extended in duration is the state of consciousness. But being conscious of consciousness is like a fish being aware of water. It is there all of the time, and we adapt to its presence and normal daily experiences rarely compel us to notice it.

According to the Loops Theory of this book, the way that the brain produces consciousness is by electric vibrations of apical dendrites. This theory of consciousness was first presented in my 2007 publication[1], and the additional details presented here are extensions of that theory. The main addition to the theory involves detailing the role of the electromagnetic fields that surround the apical dendrite.

When the apical dendrite resonates, it produces electric and magnetic fields. The electromagnetic field is one of the four fundamental forces of the universe, the others being gravity, the weak force, and the strong force. As mentioned before in this book, the resonating apical dendrite is a place where the brain produces electromagnetic waves of light. Maxwell[2], the Scottish physicist, described light as a propagating wave of electric and magnetic fields. The term *propagating* indicates that, once the wave is created, it propels itself across the vast distances of space under its own power. One way to visualize how a light wave moves itself along a straight path is to add a wave to Figure 4.1 that is produced by the electromagnetic field and moves to the right off the page. The electric part of this wave is produced by the vertically oriented field lines and the magnetic part is produced by the horizontal field circles. The electric wave looks like the resonating wave in this figure when the wave is ro-tated 90 degrees to the left and extended without end to the right. The magnetic wave has the same peaks-and-valleys appearance as the electric wave, but when it is superimposed upon the electric wave the peaks point into the page and the valleys point toward the reader (images of this com-bined wave can easily be found on the Internet). When the electric wave changes from valley to peak it causes the magnetic wave to change from valley to peak, and vice versa, endlessly. In this manner the causal link between the two fields perpetuates its movement across space.

The Near and Far Fields of Electromagnetic Vibrations

The electromagnetic wave described in the preceding paragraph radi-ates to infinity (unless absorbed or reflected). It is called the *far field* of electromagnetic light and it is illustrated by the second and third rows of drawings in Figure 11.1. The other kind of field is called the *near field* and it is illustrated by the drawings in the first row of Figure 11.1). The near field stays in contact with the apical dendrite, which is the source of the light. To understand what is happening in the near field it may help to imagine the vibrating string of a guitar or violin. When a low-pitched string is plucked, you can sometimes see the movements

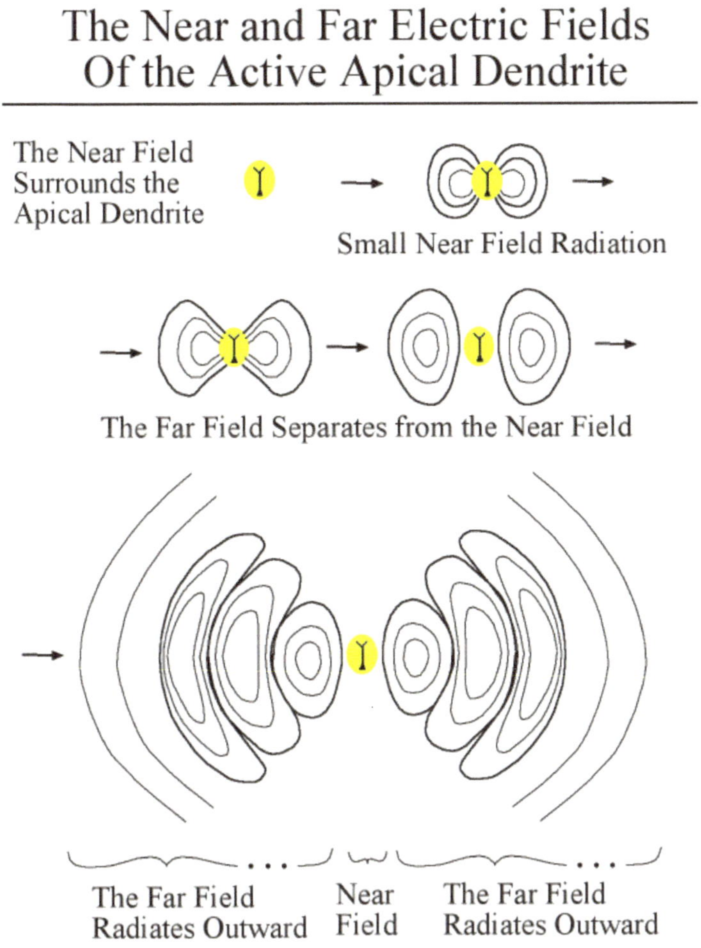

The Near and Far Electric Fields
Of the Active Apical Dendrite

The Near Field
Surrounds the
Apical Dendrite

Small Near Field Radiation

The Far Field Separates from the Near Field

The Far Field   Near   The Far Field
Radiates Outward   Field   Radiates Outward

Figure 11.1

of vibrations, and if you touch the string with your finger, you can feel a "tingle" of the string. The tingle seems to be very close to the string because you must actually touch the string to feel it. The sensation of a tingle is very brief because your finger immediately absorbs the vibration (i.e., dampens the vibration). Thus, the tingle helps us imagine what it is like to be very close to a source of a vibration in the near field.

The far field radiates waves of light which keep traveling outward from the apical dendrite as they rapidly shift from electric to magnetic and back (like the movements of two dancers) until they encounter an object that absorbs or reflects them (see Figure 11.1).

Figure 11.1 shows how the vibrating apical dendrite first produces the near field and then the near field produces the far field. The near field contains two parts: the "reactive" part (colored yellow), and the radiating part (colored grey). In the reactive part of the near field, the field lines remain in contact with the apical dendrite, and the field continues to interact with the apical dendrite. In the radiative part of the near field, the field separates from the apical dendrite, like a bubble breaks away from a wand with a circular end that has just been dipped in soapy water and someone blows air on it. The interactions between the reactive part of the near field and the apical dendrite fiber are very complex and hard to measure because the strength of the near field decays very quickly with distance from the apical dendrite (actually, the near field also contains a radiative part, but it is weaker than the reactive field).

As a consequence, the far field produces pure radiation, and the strength of the radiating field decays so slowly with distance from the apical dendrite that it never dies out. Therefore we can see radiating light from stars located at great distances from us. In view of these considerations, it is proposed here that the near field of the apical dendrite is the source of the subjective aspect of electric vibrating (resonating), and the radiating far field produces the objective aspect of resonating because it provides the way in which waves of light are observed and measured. For example, the EEG records the electromagnetic waves given off by the active brain at the scalp, which are radiated from active apical dendrites within the brain.

Therefore, when describing consciousness, it seems appropriate to separate the radiating field of light from the source of the light, and give these two aspects of light different labels. In this book, the far field is named the *wave of consciousness*, and the source in the near field is named *core consciousness*. The near field needs an object to provide the core source that generates the field of electromagnetic vibration (light) and the apical dendrite provides that object. Once the near field is produced, it produces the far field and the energy contained in it maintains its electric-to-magnetic "dance" that propels the field across space.

Waves of light are produced by candles, neon tubes, x-ray machines, by incandescent wires within light bulbs and also by resonating apical dendrites in the brain. Although the detailed composition of those waves may differ in frequency they are all waves of light that are resonating. If the vibrating field of consciousness within the brain can radiate to the outside of the brain, does this imply the reverse, namely that electromagnetic fields of consciousness outside the brain (produced from other sources) can also radiate to other locations in the inside of the brain and influence the production of other states of core consciousness within the brain? Evidence from transcranial electric and magnetic stimulation of the brain[4] indicate the beginning of an answer to this question. However, it seems important to remind ourselves that the resonating fields of clusters of apical dendrites are quite weak compared to the fields typically imposed upon them by the transcranial stimulating devices used in these experiments.

The resonating of the apical dendrite may provide a physical basis for generating consciousness in the brain, but it is not clear that waves of consciousness, once produced by the brain, can themselves influence other neural events taking place in the brain. The scarcity of proposals of how consciousness affects the brain results partly from the belief, especially among scientists, that consciousness does not exist outside of the brain. However, according to the present theory, consciousness in the form of far fields of electromagnetic vibrations does exist outside the brain, and when a sufficiently strong wave of an appropriate frequency makes contact with an apical dendrite, it presumably can cause it to vibrate and produce core consciousness within the brain in the form of near fields of electromagnetic vibrations.

A major difference between resonating consciousness inside the brain and waves of consciousness outside the brain is that resonating consciousness inside the brain begins with birth and ends with death of the body, while radiating waves of consciousness outside the brain can exist before the birth of a brain and after the death of a brain. The brain's mind can leave a record of its experiences on waves of consciousness because the far field of apical dendrite continually radiates from the inside of the brain to the outside of the brain, although at very low intensities (amplitudes). Therefore, the light wave record of our personal experience keeps moving among the many other light waves that are moving in outer space. It is intriguing to consider what could be put into the far field record of the activities of the individual brain. If the far field waves acted like radio waves, which carry the sounds of speech and music, then the informational content (in coded form) of what is happening in the mind could be part of the wave record sent into space.

Television and radio provide very instructive analogies for the production, transmission, and reception of electromagnetic waves because they are physically the same as waves from the brain when viewed at the level of waves and fields. What is different is the nature of the devices that produce and receive the fields and waves, the "dry" inorganic, hardware of electronic devices versus the "wet" organic hardware of neurons. Once launched by a television antenna or by a brain apical dendrite, they are essentially the same physical phenomenon.

However, it is not clear how the waves produced by the vibrating apical dendrite can be made to carry the coded sounds of speech and the pixels of a visual image as the waves of a television set does. Therefore, at the present state of knowledge about neural activity, it seems that the activities of network circuits would not be easily coded into a form that could enable them to be carried by the far field waves generated by apical dendrites. It seems more likely that it is the waves from apical dendrites that produce feelings and sensory impressions that are more likely to be launched into endless journeys through outer space. Could it turn out that the legacy of our lives as recorded waves of brain activity is not what we specifically said and did during our lives, but only how we felt during the saying and the doing, and how we spent our moments of time simply experiencing what we were sensing and feeling?

Let us pause here and consider what it would be like if a source (or a force) of resonating consciousness did exist outside of the physical world and it could influence what is going on in our brain. Free of (or different from) the hard cause-and-effect connections of the physical world, how would that consciousness work? How are decisions arrived at in a world of pure consciousness? And once a decision is made in consciousness, how could it be relayed back to the circuits of the brain?

The Mind-Body problem

Descartes, a philosopher living in the 17th century, wrestled with a similar problem, called the mind-body problem, and came up with the hypothesis that a tiny structure in the middle of the brain, the pineal gland, carries out the mind-to-brain transfer. Critics soon rejected this solution simply by pointing out that it still did not explain how mind stuff could affect body-stuff because it merely moved this problem to the inside of the pineal gland.

The view that the mind and body both exist as separate entities became known as mind-body dualism, and in the hundreds of years since Descartes, the solution of how they could interact with each other has remained elusive. Of course, one solution is to assert that the mind and body are not separate kinds of stuff, but either the mind is the activity of the physical body (identity theory) or the body is actually the activity of the mind (idealism). Put more informally, one could speak either of the brain's mind or the mind's brain.

There is another solution to the mind-brain problem that regards consciousness as an epiphenomenon. The epiphenomenal view of consciousness has survived many philosophical disputes over the past four centuries and remains today a reasonable solution of the mind-body problem for many serious thinkers. The epiphenomenal view regards consciousness as similar to the bell of a clock, whose sound has no role in keeping the time, or as similar to the whistle of a train that has no causal effect on the moving of the wheels of the train. In this manner, the mind, or consciousness exists in a world parallel to the physical workings of the brain, and while it is affected by the brain, it does not itself affect the workings of the brain.

In this book, consciousness is regarded as the near field of electromagnetic activity (light), and its near field is something entirely different than the computer-like movements of neuronal pulses in network circuits. Books and talk are made up of descriptions of things by using words, and it is hard to communicate new ideas about the brain without these descriptive tools. However, describing consciousness is a very different kind of event than experiencing it, and even depicting it as an electrical vibration of the apical dendrite is still only a description. We have to use other ways to communicate what is happening in the brain when we experience consciousness.

If we touch the top of a guitar or violin after one of its strings has been plucked, this direct experiencing of a vibration gives us something other than a description. This way of experiencing a vibration resembles the experiencing of "jazz" by "digging" it. We addressed this issue at the beginning of Chapter 4 with the statement, "You don't define jazz, you dig it." The point of that claim is that the brain shows us an alternative to giving a descriptive definition. Instead of trying to define "jazz" with words, you listen to it and "dig" it by slightly moving your arms and legs in rhythm to the music, and sensing how your body feels while you are doing these things.

Chapter 12

Summary and Conclusions

If one wanted to express informally the overall conclusion of this book in one sentence, that sentence might be, "The apical dendrites open doors to rooms of the mind where words do not go." We have reached that conclusion by examining two kinds of circuits in the cerebral cortex of the brain. One kind of circuit, the network circuit, is well-known because it is the basic circuit of a computer, and it "opens doors to rooms where words and numbers go." It is made up of neurons and the connections between them, in much the same way as computer circuits contain small processing devices and wires that connect them. In both the brain and the computer, these circuits are active when brief electric pulses pass along their connections. Because of this similarity between computer and brain circuits, the computer has served as a successful model for many human mental activities, such as perceiving, thinking, learning, and making decisions. Considering this history of successes, many investigators have tried to expand the computational activity of the network circuit to produce other aspects of mental life, such as having feelings and sensations. However, thinking and feeling seem to be very different kinds of mental activity to many of us, and perhaps that is because they are based on brain circuits that work in different ways and have different consequences.

In order to provide a neural framework for describing feelings and sensations, this book describes another kind of brain circuit, called the loop circuit that contains the apical dendrite. The early chapters of this book describe the structure and workings of the apical dendrite, and the chapters that follow describe applications of the loop circuit of the apical dendrite to major activities of mental life, including the production of consciousness.

The main difference between the loop circuit and the network circuit is the presence of the apical dendrite within the loop circuit. Changes in the biophysical structure (the hardware) of a circuit could change the activity of a circuit in ways that changes in programming (the software) do not. It turns out that the apical dendrite does not process information like a network neuron, but instead it vibrates electrically as pulses in the loop circuit continue to activate it. Therefore, a neuron that contains an apical dendrite can keep sending out a steady series of pulses for extended durations of time. This continuous output feature of the apical dendrite in its loop circuit contrasts with the very brief activity of network neurons, which quickly process the brief inputs of pulses into brief outputs of pulses and then is ready for the next input. For example, recognizing the color of a flower takes place very quickly, while enjoying the sensation of the color of a flower may last many seconds or even longer. In doing these things the apical dendrite employs a different kitnd of biophysical hardware, which provides a direct way to produce psychological states of feelings and sensations, and to provide ways to change the durations and intensities of experiencing them.

The ability of the apical dendrite to stay active for extended durations makes it very appropriate for producing the long periods of time of having a feeling about something or someone. The feeling of "having a good time" at a party is not a matter of one jolt of joy after another, but instead involves a continuous extension of a general state produced by apical dendrites resonating in their loop circuits. Note that the view of the brain described here does not replace the computer model of the brain, but instead adds to the computer model the simple loop circuits containing the apical dendrite which operate to give us sensations and feelings, which combine in the word *sentience*. When a yoga teacher asks you to hold a particular pose, the next words you may hear are: "Now move your attention from thinking to feeling." In the context of Loops Theory, this statement regards thinking as an activity of network circuits and feeling as an activity of loop circuits, where feelings range from intense emotion-based feelings to mild feelings of a mood.

Feelings are anchored in the body, and so we are made aware of our feelings when we listen to our bodies, particularly to the skin surfaces, and to internal organs. Neurons that specialize in specific tactual feelings are located in the somatosensory cortical area next to the back of the insula, while whole-body feelings of joy, sadness and general unease are produced by the hub-like neurons at the front of the insula. It is significant that network neurons are present in the back of the insula, but apparently absent in the front part of the insula, because the frontal insula apparently contains only apical dendrites and few, if any, network circuits.

At the neural *hub* of feelings, located in circuits of the frontal insula, many different sources of feelings come together so that when activity is sent to that hub along one spoke of the wheel, the center hub, in turn, sends this activity along all of the many other spokes to their origins. For example, when listening to or imagining a special melody builds feelings in the hub of the frontal insula, the hub then relays this activity to the body, which produce goose bumps on the surface of the skin, and to the internal organs that produce other physical expressions of emotion such as a change in heart rate.

In other words, the hub sends its intensified activity back along all of the other routes to the many brain structures that contribute to bodily feelings. No wonder that, at times like these, people report that they feel like a completely unified presence, a whole being: "This is really me, the whole me." Sensations arising from external senses of the body (seeing, hearing, tasting, smelling) are produced by apical dendrite activity in loop circuits of the primary cortical areas of these senses, where the most detailed and most vivid experiences take place. Higher areas that identify what is sensed seem to provide impressions that are less vivid, and yet they are often the targets of voluntary attention controlled by the frontal cortex. It is noteworthy that the attention control centers in the frontal cortex can directly activate the higher sensory areas of the cortex but do not directly activate the primary areas (the primary sensory areas are usually activated from voluntary frontal areas by way of higher sensory areas). It would seem that this is a good thing because direct activation of primary cortical areas by the frontal area could voluntarily distort the appearance of the environment registered in the primary sensory area and result in responses that could endanger the life of the individual.

The apical dendrite gives us the ability to attend to things. The way that the apical dendrite produces attention to an object is by increasing the intensity of the pulses in its loop circuit. When an object is not attended, as when it is in the background of a scene, each pulse consists of only one electric spike. When an object is attended, each pulse contains more than one spike, called burst firing. Low level attention is produced by bursts that contain 2 or more spikes, and a high level of attention is produced by bursts that contain 4 or more spikes, with the maximum being about 7 spikes. In this manner, attention can be adjusted to more than one level of intensity.

Increasing the intensity of pulses by burst firing can serve to select network circuits for special processing because different network circuits are activated by different loop circuits. If the pulse outputs of neurons in a particular network are increased in intensity, then these pulses will dominate the inputs from other neurons, and input pulses of lower intensities will not be accepted for processing. Also, the duration of attention to an object can easily be adjusted by how long its loop circuit is kept active. It should be noted that the choice of which object receives attention and the choice of adjusting the intensity and duration of attention are controlled by other loop circuits found in the voluntary control areas which are located in the frontal cortex of the brain.

In my 1995 book, *Attentional Processing, The Brain's Art of Mindfulness*[1], I presented a review of what was known at that time about the neural basis of three aspects of attention: selective attention, preparatory attention, and the sustaining of attention simply for its own sake. According the Loops Theory of the present book, all three of these modes of attention depend on the number of spikes in a pulse, and the last two modes of attention depend upon the duration of activity in loop circuits.

The loop circuits form the basis for learning skills and creating a sense of familiarity with objects. The gradual learning of a skill with practice and the gradual process of becoming familiar with objects, paintings, and musical tunes depends upon how many times an individual practices a skill with attention and how many times the individual observes an object with attention. Each of these occasions presents an opportunity to shift an apical dendrite from a state of potential activity to a state of brief or sustained activity. In this manner, a cluster of active apical dendrites gradually grows larger and larger. Larger clusters of apical dendrites produce higher activity from the presentation of an object and therefore a higher accuracy in performing a response to it. Chapter 7 describes brain scans of individuals while they view paintings and while they learn a skill. The brain scanning data support the claim that the higher the familiarity and the higher the level of the skill, the larger the number of active apical dendrites that are involved.

Up to this point, the benefits of the apical dendrite described in this chapter have emphasized the things that loop circuits do, such as producing sensations and feelings, and regulating the intensity and duration of attention. We turn now to the benefits of the apical dendrite to the workings of network circuits, and again we start with the computer as our model because most readers have a general idea of what it does and how it works.

Successful information processing within network circuits of computers requires that all the tiny devices (interconnected by wires of the network) produce their outputs at exactly the same time. In the brain, the clock that synchronizes the outputs of neurons is the apical dendrite, which provides a series of pulses (like the steady tick-tocks of a mechanical clock) that are evenly spaced. These pulses are transmitted as peaks in the vibrations of the membrane that surround the neurons, as shown in Figure 10.8. In this manner the apical dendrite clock provides the vibrational context in which neural communication takes place.

The way that neurons in a network circuit get on the same frequency (wavelength) is by being connected to the same apical dendrite. Each apical dendrite synchronizes its connected neurons by sending out a stream of steady pulses that make the neural membranes vibrate at a specific frequency. As a consequence, these neurons will accept pulses from other neurons if and only if their pulses are precisely synchronized with the vibration set by the controlling apical dendrites. Even a slight deviation from the vibration frequency of the receiving neuron will prevent a train of pulses from being accepted by one of these neurons.

Chapter 10 describes how the the two types of processing circuits interact. Loop circuits make contact with many network circuits by means of neural bridges. A *neural bridge* is provided by a pyramidal neuron that has a short apical dendrite. The upper part of this neuron is a dendrite that resonates, so that electric vibrations can be transmitted directly to it from the long apical dendrite that refines the variability of its frequency of vibration. The lower part of the neural bridge receives pulse inputs and sends pulse outputs, which is the mode in which neurons in a network operate. So, the lower part of the neural bridge is a part of the network circuitry. In this manner, both the loop and network circuits can be represented by one neuron, which is the short pyramidal neuron. When two neurons share the same frequency of vibration, it is the vibration of their membranes that make possible the transfer of pulse messages they send to each other. A diagram of the vibrating membranes of the two neurons is provided in Figure 10.8 to assist in understanding the way that two neurons communicate.

The apical dendrite makes possible many aspects of mental life that have extended durations, and perhaps the aspect of mental life with the longest duration is consciousness. Chapter 11 describes how every active apical dendrite produces a small electromagnetic field along its length that maintains its connection with the apical dendrite. This electromagnetic field is called the near field. When the near field is active it begins to form a duplicate field that ultimately separates from the near field core and becomes the far field. The far field then radiates outward. It is the radiating far field that gives us light that is typically observed. The core of the near field is not observable directly, which makes it very difficult to describe exactly what is going on within the near field even though much is known about the radiating far field. At the present time, more details of the workings of the near field need to be revealed before we can understand what is happening in the near field as well as we presently understand what is happening in the far field.

This book describes many ways that the mind can grow in perceiving the world and in responding to the world, both the world ouside and the world within one's own body. Examples range from increasing the familiarity of paintings and the skill of playing the piano, to increasing our ability to sense feelings in ourselves and others. In general, it appears that electric resonating is not only a part of being alive, but it gives us the experiences of joy and sorrow that make us feel more fully alive.

END

Footnotes

Footnotes

Chapter 2

1. Photograph of Mt. Rainier in Northwest Washington by Karen Povey.

Chapter 3

1. Valverdi F. Intrinsic neocortical organization: Some comparative aspects. *Neuroscience*, 1986,18, 1–23.
2. LaBerge D. Apical dendrite activity in cognition and consciousness. *Consciousness and Cognition*, 2006, 235–257.
3. Mountcastle VB. *The Cerebral Cortex*. Cambridge, MA: Harvard University Press. 1998.

Chapter 5

1. The main kinds of EEG waves are shown in Figure 4.4.
2. Yamawaki N, Shepherd GMG. (2015), Synaptic circuit organization of motor cortico-thalamic neurons. *Journal of Neuroscience*. doi:10,1523/jneurosci.4023-14.2015.

Chapter 6.

1. One spike or several closely-spaced spikes injects a mass of positive charges into the top of the apical dendrite. This surge of charges then moves down the apical dendrite to the cell body. The intensity of the surge usually is not large enough to produce a spike.

2. Hulme TE. Bergson's Theory of Art, Section 29. In Read H. *Speculations: Essays on Humanism and the Philosophy of Art*, 1924, Harcourt, Brace, Jovanovich.

3. Petersen SE, Robinson DL, and Keys, W. (1985). Pulvinar nuclei of the behaving rhesus monkey: visual responses and their modulation. *J. Neurophysiology.* 54, 867–886.

4. Rafal RD & Posner MI, Deficits in human visual spatial attention following thalamic lesions. *Proceedings of the National Academy of Science*, 1987, 7349-7353. doi: 10.1073/pnas.84.20.7349.

5. LaBerge D. and Buchsbaum MS. (1990). Positron emission tomographic measurements of pulvinar activity during an attention task. *Journal of Neuroscience*, 2, 613-619.

6. Jones, EG. (2009). Synchrony in the interconnected circuitry of the thalamus and cerebral cortex. *Annals of the New York Academy of Science*; 1157:10-23. doi: 10.1111/j.1749-6632.2009.04534.

7. Buchsbaum MS, Buchsbaum B, Chokron S, Tang C, Wei TC, Byne W. Thalamocortical circuits: fMRI assessment of the pulvinar and medial dorsal nucleus in normal volunteers. *Neuroscience Letters*. 404: 282- 287. doi.10.1016/jneulet.2006.05.063

8. Photographs and diagrams of the cortex seen in cross-section show the horizontal bands of axon fibers from cell fibers shown in Figure 10.1. The band of Baillarger contains axons of layer 5 pyramidal neurons that spread to other pyramidal neurons located in nearby columns and inhibit their activities via connections to inhibitory neurons located nearby. So, when a particular pyramidal neuron target is selected during attention it will also inhibit other pyramidal neurons that represent distracting features or objects that are similar to that pyramidal neuron target.

9. LaBerge D, Samuels SJ. (1974). Toward a theory of automatic information processing in reading. *Cognitive Psychology*, 6, 293-323. doi:org/10.1016/0010-0285(74)900152.

10. James W. (1884). The dilemma of determinism. *Unitarian Review*, 1884, 9, 193-222.

11. Eliot TS. (1950). *The Metaphysical Poets*. In *Selected Essays*. New York: Harcourt, Brace. "Tennyson and Browning are poets, and they think; but they do not feel their thoughts as immediately as the odor of a rose. A thought to Donne was an experience; it modified his sensibility. The poets of the seventeenth century, the successors of the dramatists of the sixteenth, possessed a mechanism of sensibility that could devour any kind of experience."

12. Eliot TS, (1920). *Hamlet and his Problems; The sacred wood: Essays on poetry and criticism*. London. Methuen.

Chapter 7.

1. Baudry M. Synaptic Plasticity: Learning and memory in normal aging, *Encyclopedia of Neuroscience*, (2009), 757-762. First discovered by Terje Lømo in 1966, long-term potentiation (LTP) is a long-lasting strengthening of synapses between nerve cells. Psychologists use LTP to explain long-term memories.

2. Hippocampal long term potentiation is described in Baudry M, Zhu G, Liu Y, Briz V, Bi X. (2015).*Brain Research, (*2015) 1621: 73–81. doi:10.1016/j.brainres.2014.11.033.

3. Williams LE, Holtmaat A. Higher-order thalamocortical inputs gate synaptic long-term potentiation via disinhibition. 2018.doi.org/10.1016/j.neuron.2018/10.04.

4. Boutet I, Taler V, Collin CA. (2015). On the particular vulnerability of face recognition to aging: A review of three hypotheses. *Frontiers in Psychology*, 6, 1139. doi 10.3389/fpsyg.2015.01139.

5. Elbert T, Pantev C, Wienbruch C, Rockstroh B, Taub, E. (1995). Increased cortical representation of the fingers of the left hand

in string players. *Science*, 13, 1325-1327.

6. Falk D, Lepore F, Noe A. (2013). The cerebral cortex of Albert Einstein: a description and preliminary analysis of unpublished photographs. *Brain*, 136, 1304–1327. doi:org.10.1155/2016/6817397.

7. Meier J., Topka SM, Hanggi J. (2016). Differences in cortical representation and structural connectivity of hands and feet between professional handball players and ballet dancers. *Neural Plasticity*. doi: 10.1155/2016/6817397.

8. Hyde KL, Lerch J, Norton A, Forgeard M, Winner E, Evans AC, Schlaug G. (2009). The effects of musical training on structural brain development: A longitudinal study. *Annals of the New York Academy of Sciences, 1169. The Neurosciences and Music III: Disorders and Plasticity*, 182–186.

9. Kosslyn SM, Thompson WL, Ganis G. (1994). *Image and Brain.* Cambridge, MA, MIT Press.

Chapter 8

1. Vartanian O, Skov M. Neural correlates of viewing paintings: evidence from a quantitative meta-analysis of functional magnetic resonance imaging data from 15 experiments. *Brain and Cognition*, 2014, 87, 52-56. doi: 10.1016/j.bandc.2014.03.004.

2. Cupchik GC, 2. 2. Vartanian O, Crawley A, Mikulis DJ.Contributions of cognitive control and perceptual facilitation to aesthetic experience. *Brain and Cognition*, 2009. doi.org/10.1016/j.bandc.2009.01.003.

3. van Halteren-van Tilborg IADA, Scherder EJA, Hulstijn W. Motor-Skill Learning in Alzheimer's Disease: A Review with an Eye to the Clinical Practice. *Neuropsychology Review*, 2007.17, 203–212. doi:10.1007/s11065-007-9030-14.

4. The neurotransmitter dopamine is believed to be related to reward-related learning, and originates in a region in the midbrain, known as the substantia nigra, which is a nucleus of neurons within the (subcortical) basal ganglia.

5. Bertolevo et al, 2018. A mechanistic model of connector hubs, modularity and cognitions. *Nature Human Behavior*. Vol 1, 765-767.

6. Così la mente mia, tutta sospesa,
   mirava fissa, immobile e attenta,
   e sempre di mirar faceasi accesa.
   A quella luce cotal si diventa,
   che volgersi da lei per altro aspetto
   è impossibil che mai si consenta;
   Dante. *Commedia*, Paradiso, Canto 33, lines 97-102.

7. Bierstadt A., Sunset in the Rockies.

Chapter 9 The Insula and Feelings

1. Morel A, Gallay DS. 2012. The human insula: architectonic organ-ization and postmortem MRI registration. *Neuroscience* 236, 117–135. doi: 10.1016/j.neuroscience.2012.12.076.

2. Craig, A.D. How do you feel—now? The anterior insula and human awareness. (2009). *Nature Reviews Neuroscience*. 1. 59-70. doi:10.1038/nrn2555.

3. Ishizu T. Zeki T. (2011). Toward A brain-based theory of beauty. *PLoS ONE*. doi.org10,1371/journal.pone.0021852.

4. Lutz A, Brefczynski-Lewis J, Johnstone T, Davidson RJ. (2008). Regulation of the neural circuitry of emotion by compassion meditation: effects of meditative expertise. PLoS ONE doi:10.1371/journal.pone.

5. Critchley, H. D., Wiens, S., Rotshtein, P., Ohman, A., & Dolan, R. J. (2004). Neural systems supporting interoceptive aware-ness. *Nature Neuroscience*, 7, 189–195.7.

6. Mufson EJ, and Mesulam MM. Thalamic connections of the insula in the rhesus monkey and comments on the paralimbic connectivity of the medial pulvinar nucleus. *Journal of Comparative Neurology*, 1984, doi.org/10.1002/cne.902270112. The orbital prefrontal cor-tex (OPFC) is connected with the mediodorsal (MD) nucleus and

the medial pulvinar (Pul M), nuclei of the thalamus, which in turn are connected to the frontal insula by a chain of connections.

7. Kelly.C. Torobcd R, Martino AD, Cox CL, Bellec P, F. Castellanosa FX, Milham MP. A convergent functional architecture of the insula emerges across imaging modalities. *NeuroImage*. 2012. https://doi.org/10.1016/j.neuroimage.2012.03.021.

8. Evrard HC. The Organization of the Primate Insular Cortex. *Frontiers in Neuroanatomy. 2019.* doi.org/10.3389/fnana.2019.00043.

9. Gogolla H. The insular cortex, *Current Biology*. 2017, 27, 580-585.

10. Taylor GJ Bagby R, Parker JDA. *Disorders of Affect Regulation: Alexithymia in Medical and Psychiatric Illness.* Cambridge University Press, 1999.

11. Lamm C, Singer T. The role of the anterior insula in social emotions. *Brain Structure & Function*. 2010. doi: 10.1007/s00429-010-0251-3.

12. Spagna A, Dufford AJ, Wu Q, T, ZhenW, Coons EE, Hof PR, Hu B, Wu Y, Fan J. Gray matter volume of the anterior insular cortex and social networking. *Journal of Comparative Neurology*. 2018. doi:10.1002/cne.24402.

13. Allman JM, Watson KK, Tetreault, NA, Hakeem AY. Intuition and autism: a possible role for Von Economo neurons. *Trends in Cognitive Sciences*, 2005, 9, 367-373. doi.org/10.1016/j.tics.2005.06.008_

14. Dosenbach NU, Fair DA, Miezin FM, Cohen AL, Wenger KK, Dosenbach RA, Fox MD, Snyder AZ, Vincent JL, Raichle ME, Schlaggar BL, Petersen SE. Distinct brain networks for adaptive and stable task control in humans. *Proceedings of the National Academy of Science, USA*. 2007, 104, 11073-11078.

15. Allman JM, Tetreault NA, Atiya Y. Hakeem AY. Kebreten F. Manaye, KS, Erwin JM, Park S, Goubert V, and Hof PR. (2011). The von Economo neurons in the frontoinsular and anterior cingulate cortex. doi:10.1111/j.1749-6632.2011.06011. *Annals of the New York* Academy of Science.

16. Anastassiou AC, Perin R, Markram H, and Koch C. (2011). Ephaptic coupling of cortical neurons. *Nature Neuroscience*. (2011).

17. Peters, A, Yilmaz, E. Neuronal organization in area 17 of cat visual cortex. *Cerebral Cortex*, 1993, 3, 49-68.

Chapter 10. Being on the Same Wavelength

1. The equation that relates wavelength to frequency is $f = V / L$, where f represents frequency, V represents the velocity of the wave, and L represents wavelength. So, when the velocity of the wave is constant (e g., in air, or in a copper wire, or in neural tissue), the frequency of a wave peak will be the same as 1 divided by the wavelength, and vice versa. Long wave lengths correspond to low frequencies, and short wave lengths correspond to high frequencies.

2. The exact spike rate within a burst is notoriously difficult to measure, and the range given here for the range of relatively fast firing rates of spikes within a burst should be regarded as an informal estimate.

3. Llano DA, Sherman SM, (2009). Differences in intrinsic properties and local network connectivity of identified layer 5 and layer 6 adult mouse auditory corticothalamic neurons support a dual corticotha-lamic projection hypothesis *Cerebral Cortex*, 19, 2810–2826. doi:10.1093/cercor/bhp050.

4. Mercer A, West DC, Morris OT, Kirchhecker S, Kerkhoff JJE, Thomsson AM (2005). Excitatory connections made by presynaptic cortico-cortical pyramidal cells in layer 6 of the neocortex. *Cerebral Cortex*, 15, 1485-1496. doi.org/10.1093/cercor/bhi027.

5. Sherman, SM, & Guillery, RW. 1998. On the actions that one nerve cell can have on another: distinguishing 'drivers' from 'mod-ulators'. *Proceedings of the National. Academy of Science, USA*. 1998, 95, 7121–7126. doi: 10.1073/pnas.95.12.7121.

6. Kasevich RS, LaBerge D. (2011). Theory of electric resonance in the neocortical apical dendrite. P*LoS ONE 6:e23412*. doi: 10.1016/j.concog.2013.10.004.

7. While I was a visiting instructor at Simon's Rock College (now named Bard College at Simon's Rock) from 1998 to 2008, Ray attended my

classes. Ray's field of expertise is electrical physics, and he directs the Stanley Laboratory of electrical physics in Great Barrington, MA, which engages in research for a variety of companies worldwide. His laboratory is located close to Bard College at Simon's Rock, where Ray now teaches courses in the electrical physics of neurons. The close proximity of his laboratory to the college made it easy for us to have weekly meetings in his office during which he extended my knowledge of electrical physics and I extended his knowledge of cognitive neuroscience. We collaborated in 4 publications.

8. Delogne P. *Leaky Feeders and Subsurface Radio Communication.* New York: Peter Peregrinus, *1982.*

9. The equation given by Delogne is based on a leaky cable model of the neuron (the apical dendrite has many pores through which chemical charges pass), and the parameter values for the electrical properties of the neuron were taken from recent neurophysiological publications. The aim of the mathematical model was to see what the movement of current down the apical dendrite would do to the surges of electric charges that entered the first compartment of the apical dendrite. The axon pulses entering at the top of the apical dendrite (the first compartment) will typically produce surges having a range of frequencies, which can be described as a profile or distribution of frequencies. With the basic equation in hand, the energy transfer value (maximum) from the first to the second compartment was calculated for 4 specific regulating frequencies, 20, 40, 60, and 80 Hz (cycles per second), using an iterative procedure. With each value of energy transfer it was then possible to calculate how rapidly positive charges (of potassium ions) leak out through the membrane channels. This outward movement of potassium ions turns out to be the way that the apical dendrite regulates the frequency of pulses in the loop circuit of which it is a part.

10. In a 1992 study[12] with two graduate students at the University of California, Irvine I wrote difference equations for a simulation of

activity of the thalamus-to-cortex loop circuit. This equation de-scribed how the activity level in the loop changed with each cycle of pulses around the loop circuit. The loop circuit in that model did not contain the apical dendrite because, at that time it was be-lieved that the apical dendrite was simply another dendrite which summed or integrated its many input pulses to produce output pulses in the axon.

The model of the loop circuit in the 1992 study included the known inhibitory connections within the thalamus. The results of the simulation showed that when input from the location of a target is slightly larger than the input from a neighboring location, the circuit substantially increased the difference in neuron output at the target location compared with the neuron output at the neigh-boring location. Apparently, the loop circuits of two different but close locations of an object can be made more distinct by the oper-ations of the loop circuit itself.

11. LaBerge D, Carter M, and Brown, V.(1992). A network simulation of thalamic circuit operations in selective attention. *Neural Com-putation*. 1992. 4, 318-331. doi:10.1162/neco.1992.4.3.318·

12. The "vibration of a neuron" refers not only to the electric vibration of the neural core but also to the vibration of the membrane that covers all the parts of a neuron except the axon.

13. The large image in Figure 10.8 shows a cell body with only two basal dendrites connected to it (for clarity). Typically, the cell body sprouts several more basal dendrites, for example, the short pyramidal neuron of the human shown in Figure 3.1 contains about 10 basal dendrites. On the outside of the neuron shown in Figure 10.8 is a membrane whose vibration frequency is con-trolled by the apical dendrite, which is located at the top of the cell body. The voltage intensity of the membrane vibration does not reach the level needed to produce a neural spike. Hence, the vibration intensity in the membrane is regarded as subthreshold.

The thickness of the membrane in Figure 10.8 is greatly magnified to show more details of the electric plus-to-minus changes that produce the electric vibration of the membrane.

The single axon that exits at the base of the cell body sends out pulses that are timed to occur by the electrical vibration in the membrane surrounding the cell body. Each positive peak in the vibration provides the extra voltage "push" at the axon hillock that sends out a spike in the axon. Each pause between the axon spikes corresponds to the number of vibration peaks that do not result in a spike in the axon.

Whether or not the "push" of a vibration peak produces an axon output spike depends on how high the momentary activity (voltage) is in the cell body. The total momentary activity in the cell body is produced by the sum of the momentary inputs to the cell body from all of its dendrites. If the basal dendrites momentarily activate the cell body with enough strength (voltage) then the added push of activity from the ongoing vibration of the apical dendrite will be enough to produce a spike in the axon. The "trigger" that sends a spike from the cell body into the output axon is produced by a small capsule-like shape at the bottom of the cell body, which is called the axon hillock.

Therefore, the spikes and pauses produced in the output axon can form a temporal code (a time interval-based spike code) by which one neuron communicates with other neurons. The code is "carried" on the vibration frequency set by the apical dendrite and keeps going regardless of whether or not axon inputs enter the basal dendrites. Using a analogy of a radio, the receiving neuron can only "hear" the message if the receiving neuron is tuned to the same frequency as the sending neuron.

Figure 10.8 also shows how the receiving neuron can be activated by a coded message that is carried by an incoming axon. The axon input enters at the bottom left corner of the figure, and its coded message is displayed under a small part of the membrane of the basal dendrite shown on the left side of the cell body. The spikes in this coded message occur at precisely the same time as a positive peak in the membrane vibration. A spike contacts the vibrating membrane of the receiving neuron at a synapse, and the energy of the synaptic discharge and in the membrane wave sum to produce a surge of voltage shown inside the basal dendrite. This surge of voltage then moves into the cell body and sums with the voltage surges from other basal dendrites (not shown here). If the spikes of an axon input do not match the positive peak of the membrane voltage, then they will not produce current surges in the basal dendrite at a synapse.

The precision of this matching process seems less amazing when it is noted that the tiny tip of a spike will activate a synapse of the basal dendrite only if it arrives at precisely the same moment that the vibration wave of the dendrite membrane is at its positive peak (the sharp tip of a spike can be seen in Figure 6.1). If an axon spike misses a vibration peak in the membrane by even a slight amount then its voltage will not open the channel in the synapse of the membrane.

If the incoming axon spikes are to arrive at the times of the receiving neuron's vibration peaks then the vibration waves in the membrane of the sending neuron must possess the same frequency (peaks per second) as the vibration waves of the receiving neuron. If the incoming axon spikes are from a neuron that vibrates at a different frequency than that of the receiving neuron then the voltage energy of its incoming spikes cannot open a synapse of the neuron's basal dendrites, and there will be no spike energy sent at that moment to the cell body to increase the momentary intensity at the axon hillock.

14. Fries P. (2015). Rhythms for cognition: Communication through coherence. *Neuron*, 88, 220-235. doi:10.1016/j.neuron.2015.09.034.

15. The present form of Loops Theory assumes that frequency matching of the incoming series of axon spikes to the dendrite vibration is necessary and sufficient for acceptance of a series of synaptic inputs to the neuron. The phase relations between surges of current

at the dendrite-to-cell body junctions affect the momentary summation of charges in the cell body, which determines the timing of axon spikes sent from the axon hillock. In this manner, summation of phase-related dendritic inputs to the cell body can describe neural integration within the neuron.

Chapter 11. Consciousness
1. LaBerge D, & Kasevich RS. The apical dendrite theory of consciousness. *Neural Networks.* 2007, 20,1004-2020. doi: 10.1016/j.neunet.2007.09.006.
2. Maxwell JC, A dynamical theory of the electromagnetic field. *Philosophical Transactions of the Royal Society of London.*1865, 155, 459-512DOI:10.1098/rstl.1865.0008.
3. Each move in the direction of the wave trajectory requires a small interval of time, and Maxwell used his four famous equations to calculate the velocity of the coupled electric and magnetic field across space. His theoretical result was 186,000 miles per second, which is the measured speed of light.
4. Ekhtiari H, Tavakoli H, Addolorato G, et al. (2016). Transcranial electrical and magnetic stimulation (tES and TMS) for addiction medicine: A consensus paper on the present state of the science and the road ahead. *Neuroscience and Biobehavioral Reviews.* 2019, 104, 118-140. doi.org/10.1016/j.neubiorev.2019.06.007.

Chapter 12 Conclusions and Summary
1. LaBerge D. (1995). *Attentional Processing: The Brain's Art of Mindfulness.* Cambridge, MA. Harvard University Press.

Book Figure Credits and Permissions

Photograph of the author (2020), courtesy of Mike Waller.

Figure 2.1. Mt. Rainier, photograph by Karen Povey, by permission.

Figure 4.3. Photograph of a person wearing an EEG cap. Cognionics, San Diego ,CA, by permission of Mike Chi, CEO.

Figure 6.3. Photograph of a cat by Gundala Vogel. Pixabay free photos.

Figure 8.5. Painting: *Sunset in the Rockies*, by Albert Bierstadt. Public domain.

Figure 4.4. Types of Brain Waves(EEGs). Penfield W, Jasper HH. (1954). *Epilepsy and the Functional Anatomy of the Human Brain*. London, Little Brown and Co.

Figure 6.4. MRI photograph of a cross-section of the thalamus of one of the participants in a brain scan experiment by LaBerge D, Buchsbaum, M. (1990). Positron emission tomographic measurements of pulvinar activity during an attention task. 10, 613-619, *Journal of Neuroscience*, 10, 613-619.

Graphs of data from published experiments (public domain):
Figures 7.8, 7.9, 8.1, 8.2, 10.3.

The drawings of the remaining 45 figures were made by the author.

Index

alexithymia, 112, 168

alpha waves, 32

amygdala, 108, 111, 113

anterior cingulate area, 114

apical dendrite, vii, viii, ix, 12-25, 27-35, 37-38, 41-45, 47, 48, 54, 57-59, 60-67, 69-75, 79, 83-84, 87-89, 91, 92, 96-103, 108-111, 116-118, 122-123, 125-128, 130-132, 135-139, 141-146, 147-148, 150-154, 155-161, 163, 164, 169, 170, 171, 172, 174

attention, x, 45, 47-64, 70, 71, 73, 74, 91, 92, 94, 96, 97-103, 108-110, 113, 114, 125, 131, 132, 135-137, 147, 157-159, 164, 171, 175

automatic processing, 63

axon, 7, 11, 17, 20, 23, 24, 38, 40, 42, 43, 57, 61, 63, 76, 108, 114, 118, 122, 125, 126, 128, 131, 136, 138, 142-146, 164, 170-173

binding, 141

bridge, 137, 138, 139, 140, 141, 142, 146, 160

bridge neuron, 140, 142

bundle, 58, 59, 98, 99, 116, 118

burst, 48, 51, 57, 63, 66, 70, 73, 102, 110, 118, 122, 125, 135, 136, 158, 169

burst firing, 48, 51, 63, 73, 110, 122, 125, 135, 136, 158

carrier frequency, 120
cerebral cortex, 18, 70, 155, 163, 164, 166, 168, 169
circuit board, 3, 5
clock, x, 66, 121, 122, 128, 131, 145, 154, 165
cluster, 37, 38, 54, 58, 69, 70, 79, 97, 100, 101, 116, 117
cluster of apical dendrites, 37, 38, 54, 58, 69, 70, 79, 97, 100, 101, 116, 117
column, 125, 140, 164
computation, 5, 121, 128, 131, 171
consciousness, x, 147-154, 156, 161, 163, 174
context, 9, 20, 38, 74, 112, 132, 134-136, 138, 157, 160
core consciousness, 151, 152
cortex, 16, 18, 20, 32, 35, 37, 38, 40, 42, 43, 52, 57, 63, 70, 73, 75, 76, 79, 80, 83, 84, 87, 96, 97, 100, 102, 103, 105, 108, 109, 114, 125, 135, 138, 155, 158, 159, 163, 164, 166, 167, 168, 169, 170

Dante, 83, 101, 167
Delogne, 127, 170
dig, 27, 35, 154
dipole, 38, 39, 40, 79
disinhibition, 165
Divine Comedy, 83, 101

EEG, 30, 32, 35, 37, 38, 66, 150, 163, 175
EEG waves, 32, 163
electric dipole, 38, 39, 79
electric surges, 23
electric vibration, 22-24, 27, 29, 65, 108, 110-111, 116, 127, 138, 140, 147, 160, 171
electroencephalograph (EEG), 30, 32, 35, 37, 38, 66, 150, 163, 175
electromagnetic field, 28, 32, 38, 147, 151, 161, 174
electromagnetic radiation, 29, 30, 148

Eliot, T.S., 87, 88, 165
empathy, 111-113
ephaptic coupling, 116, 168
epiphenomenon, 154

far field, 148, 150, 151, 152153, 161
feelings, x, 2, 11-12, 27, 35, 52, 54, 57, 75, 88-89, 91-92, 94, 96-97, 98,
    105, 112, 113, 147, 157, 159,
free will, 64-67
frequency, 30-32, 54, 55, 111, 116, 118, 120-128, 130-136, 140-142,
    146, 151, 152, 160, 169, 170-173
frequency profile, 127, 128, 130
frequency range, 32
frontal insula, 107-114, 157, 167,

gamma waves, 32
grey matter, 20
grid, 5, 6, 9, 11, 35, 40

hard determinism, 66, 67
hippocampus, 73
hub, 110-111, 114, 157, 167,
hub circuit, 110

idealism, 153
identity theory, 153
inhibit, 45, 61, 63, 164,
insula, 52, 105-114, 157, 167
intense attention, 91
intense experience, 91, 100, 101, 103, 105

jazz, 27, 35, 154

Kasevich, Ray, vii, viii, 126, 131, 169, 174

lateral inhibition, 61
length of the apical dendrite, 12, 14, 30, 35, 47, 127, 130,
long apical dendrite, 14, 16, 110, 122, 126, 130, 132, 135, 141, 160
long-term potentiation (LTP), 165
loop circuit, 16-18, 22, 24-25, 28, 35, 37, 40, 45, 48, 49, 52, 57, 59, 60,
    62, 64-67, 69, 72, 74, 84, 88, 91, 92, 96-100, 102, 105, 108, 110,
    111, 117, 122, 125-127, 130, 132, 135-141, 145-147, 156-160, 170-
    171
Loops Theory, 110, 113, 138, 140, 157

magnetic resonance image (MRI), 52, 80, 84, 92, 109, 167, 175
magneto-encephalograph (MEG), 35, 79
Maxwell, 148, 174
memory cluster, 87, 103
mind-body problem, 153, 154
minicolumn, 116, 122, 123, 125, 126, 135, 140
motor area, 42, 45, 84, 87
Mozart, 83
myelin, 20

near field, 148, 150-152, 154, 161,
network, 6, 7, 9, 10, 11, 16-17, 18, 20, 24-25, 35, 27, 40, 42, 43, 45, 64,
    66, 69, 73, 88, 97, 100, 105, 107, 108, 111, 112, 113, 118, 121, 122,
    130, 131, 132, 134, 135-141, 145, 146, 147, 152, 154, 155-160, 168,
    169, 171, 174
network circuit, 10, 16-17, 24-25, 40, 43, 45, 66, 69, 73, 88, 97, 105,
    112, 132, 134, 135-141, 145, 147, 152, 154, 155-160
network grid, 6, 9, 11, 35, 40
neural binding, 141
neural bridge, 141, 160

neurogenesis, 75, 79, 103

neuron, vii, viii, ix, x, 5, 7-9, 11-20, 23-24, 31, 40, 42, 45, 47-48, 51, 57-58, 61, 63, 64, 70, 73, 75, 76, 79, 84, 92, 97, 102, 103, 105, 107-111, 114-123, 125-128, 130-132, 135-139, 140-146, 152, 155-161, 163, 164, 165, 166, 168, 169, 170, 171, 172, 173, 174

objective correlative, 87, 88

orbitofrontal area, 110, 114

orbitofrontal cortex, 109

oscillation, 23

pineal gland, 153

pulvinar, 52, 164, 167, 175

pyramidal neuron, 12, 14, 16, 20, 24, 38, 47, 57, 58, 61, 63, 70, 73, 75, 79, 84, 92, 102, 103, 105, 107-111, 114-116, 118, 122, 125, 128, 135, 138, 140, 141, 142, 144, 145, 146, 160, 164, 171

regular firing, 48, 122, 125, 135

resonance, 23, 30, 80, 83, 127, 130, 166, 169

resonance curve, 127, 130

resonance profile, 130

resonate, 25, 29, 30, 54, 121, 141, 147, 160

resonating, 24, 28, 29, 32, 35, 37, 39, 48, 58, 64, 66, 67, 101, 102, 111, 125, 126, 130, 141, 142, 148, 150, 151, 152, 153, 157, 161

sensibility, 88-89, 165

sentience, 11, 157

short apical dendrite, 14, 16, 73, 130, 132, 138, 139, 141, 142, 143, 160

skill, 64, 69, 73, 75, 80, 87, 100, 159, 161, 166

social awareness, 114

social networking, 112-113, 118-119, 168

soft determinism, 66

somatosensory (touch), 107, 157

spike, 7, 9, 11, 20, 23-25, 48, 57, 70, 108, 122, 125-126, 131, 135, 142-145, 158-159, 164, 169, 171-173

state, 24, 30, 32, 58, 65, 105, 109, 112, 114, 147, 151, 152, 156, 157, 159, 174

stellate neuron, 12 14, 16, 105, 107, 122, 123

surge, 20, 23, 29, 38, 126-128, 131, 142-145, 164, 170, 173

surges of current, 20, 23, 126-128, 145, 173

sympathy, 111-112

thalamus, 16, 17-21, 28, 38, 39-44, 49, 51-53, 57, 60, 62, 70, 72, 74, 84, 97, 98, 99, 100, 108, 117, 130, 135-137, 139, 164, 167, 170, 171, 175

theory of loop circuits, 48, 111

topic, vii, 2, 74, 131, 132, 135

vibration, ix, 23, 24, 27, 29, 65, 108, 110, 111, 116, 122, 125, 127, 131, 132, 136-146, 147-154, 160, 161, 171-173

Von Economo Neuron (VEN), 114-119, 168

wave of consciousness, 151

wavelength, 119-125, 131, 137, 160, 169

white matter, 20

Wright, Frank Lloyd, 83